Labyrinth of Birth

Creating a Map, Meditations and Rituals
for your Childbearing Year

by Pam England

SEVEN GATES MEDIA
Albuquerque, New Mexico

Seven Gates Media©2010 by Pam England

Artwork and illustrations©2008 & 2009 by Pam England

Meditating Woman™ and Opening the Body Labyrinths™
designed by Aja Oishi©2009

For information or permissions, contact: sevengatesmedia@gmail.com,
Albuquerque, New Mexico

sevengatesmedia.com

Printed by Bang Printing, Brainerd, Minnesota
Cover by Angela Werneke of River Light Media, Santa Fe

Library of Congress Cataloging-in-Publication Data
England, Pam
Labyrinth of Birth: Creating a Map, Meditations and Rituals for Your Childbearing Year
ISBN 978-1-61623-037-1 (pbk)

1. Pregnancy 2. Meditation 3. Labyrinth 4. Spirituality

This book is dedicated to

the wise ancestors in whose footsteps we follow;

and to all new parents finding their way through the labyrinth of birth.

What's Within the Labyrinth of Birth

Introduction

T HE LABYRINTH IS AN ANCIENT, UNIVERSAL SYMBOL representing our journey through life, ordeals and transitions. Its single, convoluted pathway begins at the opening, leads directly to the center and out again. The journey into the labyrinth's center is symbolic of letting go and of death (psychic or physical), and the journey from the center out of the labyrinth represents birth and rebirth. Walking or finger-tracing a labyrinth invokes a sensation of turning inward then outward, perhaps reminding us of our first journey from our mother's body into the world.

Archeologists are uncertain how old the labyrinth symbol is because the earliest ones may have been drawn in earth or made with rocks or rope and did not withstand the test of time. All over the world, labyrinths have been found carved in walls, stone, tombs, painted on wood and pottery, and woven into baskets and blankets. The oldest known labyrinth, a petroglyph engraving in Goa (India), is believed to be four thousand years old. Another early labyrinth, carved in a stone wall of a Neolithic tomb in Sardinia, an island in the Mediterranean Sea off the coast of Italy, is estimated to be 3500 years old. In this book you will learn how labyrinths have long been used as a tool to facilitate meditation, exemplify emergence and hero myths and to support rituals and easing childbirth.[1]

Many years ago a friend gifted me with a quirky vintage hat she found at a yard sale. A thick, gold spiral cord adorned the hat's short, flat crown. Knowing I liked to teach from stories and metaphors, she thought the hat would make an interesting teaching prop for my childbirth classes. It reminded her of an African birth teaching she'd heard about in which new mothers are told that the baby begins its birth journey in the center of the spiral, which represents the womb, and during the course of labor, it follows the rings in the spiral until it tumbles out. Some babies come quickly because there are few turns in their short spiral; other labors take longer because the baby's spiral has more circles going round and round. Little did I realize at the time that that gold spiral-hat was my introduction to some of the ancient and sacred geometric symbols of birth. For many years, that old hat hung on the wall in my teaching space.

About five years later I had my first encounter with an outdoor classic labyrinth. I was leading a workshop at a retreat space in Ohio. In the large field behind the space was a circular path lined with rocks. I saw someone walking in circles within it at sunset and asked my host what she was doing, what "it" was for. "It's a labyrinth," she answered with dispassion, "You're supposed to walk the path to the center." She guessed it was for meditation or that walking in circles would help to think things through. I walked the path to the center, then, not knowing what to do next, walked over the paths to leave. I wondered what it was all about. I didn't have a particularly memorable experience; in fact, I didn't get it at all. And thus began my search.

When I learned about the labyrinth, and after I experienced it as a meditation, I saw it as the perfect symbol or "map" of a hero's journey and of a woman's emotional and physical journey through pregnancy, labor and postpartum. Immediately, I began to introduce the labyrinth to childbirth classes and workshops.

The meandering labyrinth offers a superior alternative to explaining labor in terms of "stages of labor." The convoluted pathway more accurately portrays a mother's inner experience of labor and postpartum than does the straight line on a labor graph. Whereas the labor graph ends abruptly with the birth of the baby, the labyrinth illustrates the continuum of a mother's social, physical and spiritual journey throughout the childbearing year.

Parents experienced in birth, without exception, enthusiastically confirm that their internal experience of labor and postpartum was exactly like moving through a labyrinth. Encouraged by the lively dialogues that accompanied making labyrinths in class, I began to add two important symbols to the labyrinth drawing: the

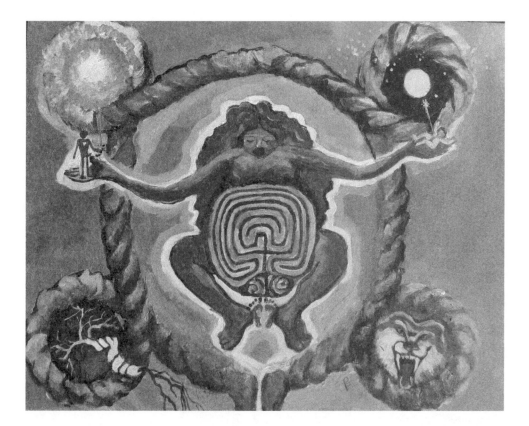

Threshold and Footprints (which are described later in this book). Over time we began referring to this unique labyrinth as a Laborinth™.

Labyrinth of Birth answers the growing yearning among new parents for ceremony and personal growth during the childbearing year. In the *Labyrinth of Birth* you will learn about childbirth labyrinths, labyrinth myths, and fourteen simple meditations and ceremonies that will enhance your childbearing year. In this book, you will learn how labyrinths have been used for centuries as a tool to facilitate meditation and to gain insight or answers to dilemmas and our deepest questions, and how they have been used in rituals for healing and initiation.

There is even a tradition of using labyrinths specifically for healing and meditation in childbirth. Here is an example: Five hundred years ago, English midwives and healers in Cornwall used labyrinths to guide them in their healing work. When people came to them with questions about life or in search of healing, the midwife would hold the patient's question in mind, and hum while tracing with her finger a labyrinth etched in slate. Tracing the labyrinth drew the midwife into a receptive, intuitive state of mind where she could see what was needed for healing. When the midwife died, it was customary to either pass her labyrinth down to her apprentice or to bury it with her.

This book is an invitation to follow in the footsteps of our ancestors and participate in the timeless tradition of making and meditating on the labyrinth. Let's get started!

Peace,

Pam England

Albuquerque, New Mexico

September 13, 2009

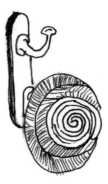

P.S. A note about why certain words are capitalized in this book. Words like Number, Center or Laborinth are capitalized when they refer to an archetype or symbol rather than the noun.

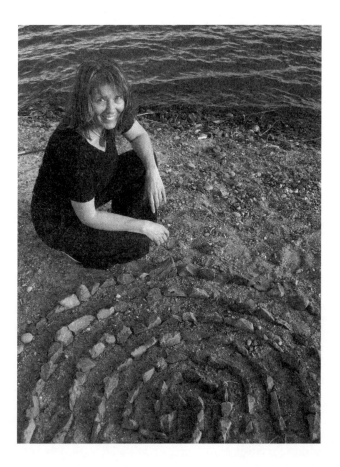

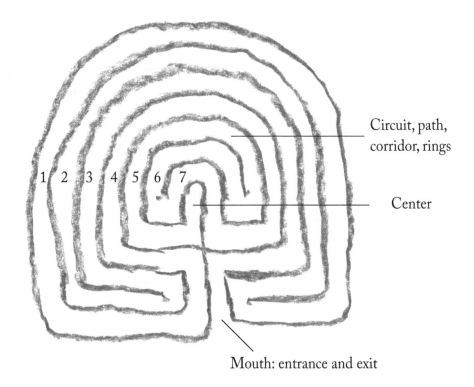

Circuit, path,
corridor, rings

Center

Mouth: entrance and exit

A CLASSIC SEVEN-CIRCUIT LABYRINTH

The seven-circuit labyrinth is referred to as the "classic labyrinth" because it is the one most widely used around the world. The Hindu yantra, the square and round Hopi labyrinths, and the Tohono O'dham nation's Man in the Maze are all seven-circuits.

Anatomy and Glossary
of a Labyrinth

U NDERSTANDING A FEW TERMS and the structure of labyrinths will enhance your enjoyment of this book.

Labyrinth: There are many variations of labyrinths. Some are small enough to fit on a coin, like the ones made in Crete (3 B.C.E.), others are big enough to cover a hill or to make a meandering path through a garden. They all share one thing in common: they are unicursal, which means there is a single path from the opening of the labyrinth to the center and back out again. There are no cul-de-sacs or dead ends.

Mouth: With a single path, there is only one entrance, which also serves as the exit: the mouth.

Circuits: Labyrinths are described by the number of their circuits, i.e. a three-circuit, seven-circuit, eleven-circuit labyrinth, and so on. The number of circuits is determined by counting the rings or paths, beginning with the outside path and counting toward the inner-most path, without counting the center.

Classification: Labyrinths are referred to by their number of circuits, geometric pattern, shape, location or time period (e.g., round, square, animal, Roman or Chartres).

Laborinth™: It's not a misspelling. "Laborinth" is coined word that refers to the unique labyrinth drawn as a map or representation of the childbearing year; it includes Footprints, a Threshold and other personal symbols.

Seed: For centuries labyrinths have been reproduced and drawn from patterns called "seeds." Check out the labyrinth seeds in the Appendix.

Maze: The word "maze" is derived from an old English word *mazen*, which means to bewilder or confuse. People often confuse a labyrinth with a maze, or think they are the same thing.

WHAT'S THE DIFFERENCE BETWEEN A LABYRINTH AND A MAZE?

The labyrinth is a single path from the mouth to the center and out again, so you can't get lost in it and you don't need to think to find your way through it. On the other hand, a maze may have more than one entrance and exit, and it has dead ends and cul-de-sacs, so you do have to think, plan and often retrace your path to find your way through and out. Modern birth can seem like a maze, which explains why so many modern mothers try to think and plan their way through labor.

In the palace at Knossos on the island of Crete, the *labrys*, double-headed axe, was a tool, a weapon in war and an important symbol as the axe was used in the ceremonial slaying of bulls. This *labrys* maze pattern was found carved in a cave wall a few miles from the palace, and it was also engraved on stone pillars and painted on the wall of the palace.[1]

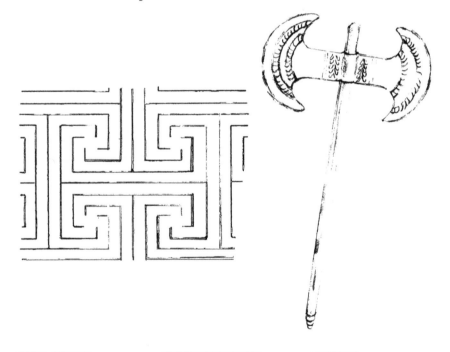

The Significance of Numbers

Whenever you see a number in ancient art, stories or sacred geometry, whether it is three, seven, twelve or any specific number, it may not be referring to the actual quantity. The ancients used Numbers as symbols to communicate complex ideas rather than quantity.

Three is associated with creation; past/present/future; crone/mother/maiden; and birth/life/death. In fairytales you find three wishes, three pigs, three brothers. Three represents Masculine energy.

Four represents manifestation, earth, completeness. This Number is found in the Four Directions, four elements (earth, fire, water, air); and in both square labyrinths and round labyrinths that have four quarters. Four represents Feminine energy.

Seven is the vibration of, and the symbol for, Mystery. It represents learning, wisdom, completion, stoicism, determination, enduring hardship and fighting without faltering. There are many examples of Seven: seven major planets, seven notes in a scale, seven chakras, seven days of the week and seven dwarves in Snow White.

Joshua and his men marched around Jericho for Seven days with Seven priests blowing Seven trumpets, the city fell on the Seventh day.[2] (See the City of Jericho labyrinth on page 2.)

Meanings of Geometrical Shapes

Labyrinths are circular, square, octagonal, and animal shapes, but most are circular.

Spiral: Cosmic energy, sun, birth, death and rebirth.

Circular: Spirit, a symbol of eternity, the shape of the sun and moon.

Square: Earth, body.

Octagon: Rebirth, renewal, infinity and transition.

Triangle: Pointing downward symbolizes water, mother, womb and the Feminine.

Pointing upward represents fire, mountain, father and the Masculine.

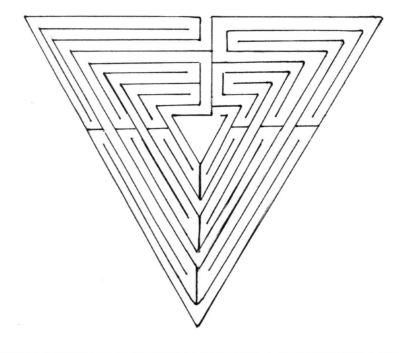

Labyrinths

from Around the World

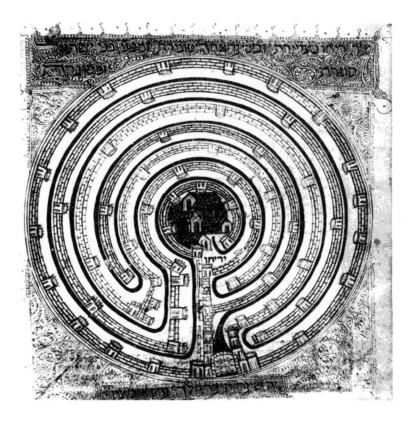

THE CITY OF JERICHO LABYRINTH

Drawn in 14th century by Elisha ben Avraham Crescas on parchment in the Farhi Bible, Spain. This labyrinth has six circuits to make seven walls. Over the entrance is a closed gate. The "road" through the labyrinth is blue in color. The walls are constructed of three layers of stone, fortified with towers. The city of Jericho is in the center, represented by several buildings.[1]

Labyrinths
from Around the World

THE LABYRINTH IS AN ANCIENT, UNIVERSAL SYMBOL representing our journey through life, ordeals and initiations. Its unicursal, convoluted pathway is associated with birth and spiritual rebirth. The journey into the labyrinth's center is symbolic of death (psychic or physical), and the journey out of the labyrinth represents birth or rebirth.

More labyrinths (over 600) have been found in Scandinavia than anywhere else in the world. Labyrinths made of stone and boulders were built near shorelines to protect sailors in two ways: It was believed that the labyrinths "captured' violent winds before they could harm ships; and, before heading out to sea, fishermen walked the labyrinth seven times so that bad spirits or trolls attached to them would be trapped in the center before they headed out to sea.[2]

Every culture has made the labyrinth uniquely their own. In China, labyrinths made from incense were used to keep time in ceremonies. New scents were introduced at the corners where the path changed direction. By noticing the new scent they knew what time it was![3]

In Medieval Europe, it was common to go to Jerusalem to walk and pray where Jesus walked and prayed. When it became too dangerous and expensive to go to Jerusalem on pilgrimmage, the church ordered seven cathedrals to build labyrinths. Mosaic labyrinths were embedded in floors of European cathedrals. Devout seekers who could not make the pilgrimage to the Holy Land made their pilgrimage by crawling on their knees through the labyrinth in the church. The center of the church labyrinths was called "Jerusalem." Unfortunately, for a while labyrinths fell out of favor with the church and many were destroyed. The most famous surviving labyrinth is in the Chartres Cathedral in France.

Tapu'at: Mother and Child

Hopi have two labyrinths, one is square, and the other is round; both are seven-circuits. Hopi are Native American people who live in northeastern Arizona. Their square labyrinth is called Tapu'at (Mother-child). It is unique because it has two entrances and contains two labyrinths, one within the other.

Tapu'at is referred to as "Mother and Child" because the outer labyrinth holds the inner labyrinth, like a mother holding her child. This labyrinth is like the mother's womb enveloping the unborn baby. The unattached center line emerging from the entrance of Tapu'at represents the umbilical cord. "Its two ends symbolize the two stages of life—the unborn child within the womb of Mother Earth, and the child after it is born. The "u" shaped lines on the outer edges represent the fetal membranes which enfold the child within the womb. The outside lines represent the mother's arms which hold the child later."[4]

Tapu'at also represents emergence and spiritual rebirth from one world to the succeeding one. The passages through the round labyrinth represent the plan of the Creator which humans must follow on their road of life.

To experience this labyrinth, enter the upper "mouth" (the mother path) and trace the left path, then enter the lower "mouth" (the child path) and trace the right path.

The Hopi round labyrinth is a classic seven-circuit, but its design and meaning differ from the square one. The center line at the entrance, which is connected in the typical way, symbolizes the Sun Father, the giver of life, the seed of life that penetrates the womb. The four points represent the Four Directions. This labyrinth is included in Hopi ceremonies.[5]

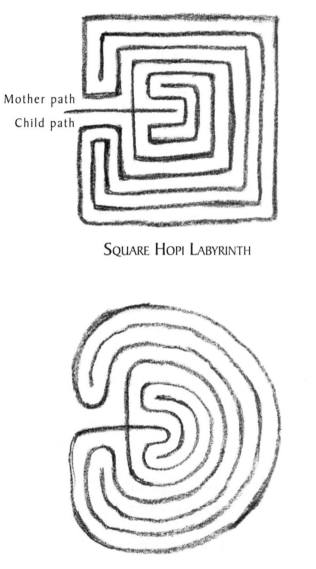

Mother path

Child path

SQUARE HOPI LABYRINTH

ROUND HOPI LABYRINTH

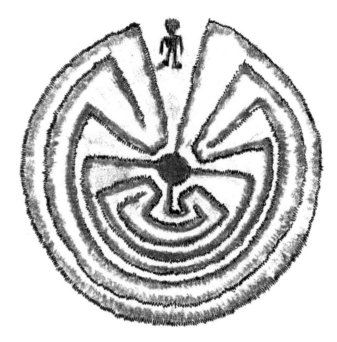

Man in the Maze

MAN IN THE MAZE was designed by the Tohono O'odham Nation (formerly called Papago) in the Central Valley of Arizona. In the early 1900s they began weaving this unique seven circuit labyrinth into their baskets using desert plants, dried leaves, stems and roots.

"Man in the Maze" represents their Emergence myth. The round layers represent the womb; the male figure standing in the entrance may represent the human seed entering the womb, fertilization, gestation and emergence in birth. It also symbolizes life and choice: "right" choices lead us to harmony even when the road is long. The dark center suggests we journey from darkness into light; it also represents a person's unlived dreams, goals, and the next world.[6]

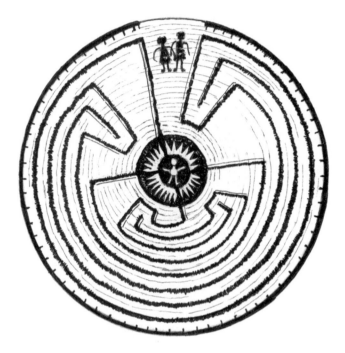

This "Family in the Maze" design was woven in a basket made with pink and black yarn. The basket was found in a garage sale, so I don't know who made it or from where it came. Perhaps it is a recent design developed for tourists.

Childbirth Yantras

A YANTRA IS A UNIQUE KIND OF LABYRINTH FROM INDIA. Yantra is a Sanskrit word: "yan" means support, "tra" refers to an instrument. For two thousand years, yantras have been used in India to focus attention, eliminate mind chatter and deepen meditation. There are many variations in the colorful, geometric designs of yantras, and each one contains layers of symbolic relevance. They are usually drawn on gold, silver, copper, paper and the earth, however, certain yantras used in healing are drawn directly on the body of the patient.[7]

The sacred geometric design of the yantra helps sustain and support the energy of a certain idea. This instrument helps the mother visualize and hold the image of the baby moving from her womb into the world. So, when a woman is in labor, Hindu midwives hang a yantra on the wall of her birth room and encourage her to gaze upon the yantra while using her own mental powers to assist the birth.

The yantra is hung on a wall facing north or east. The center of the yantra should be at eye level. In the center of many yantras is a black dot on a white background (bindi), which represents the principle of manifestation, the origin of unity. In one yantra meditation, the mind concentrates on this single point—while seeing the whole yantra.

When gazing upon her childbirth yantra (labyrinth), the mother may rest her eyes softly on the center while taking in the whole yantra. Or, she may follow the labyrinthine path with her eyes, from the opening to the center and out again, during or in-between contractions, "showing her baby the way out." She may also focus on a word or mantra to further focus and calm her mind. The intense concentration required to do this in labor calms the mother's breath and mind, thereby easing the pain. In the meditative state of mind she can more easily access her intuitive knowing.

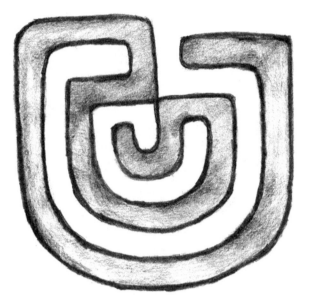

ABHYUMANI YANTRA

A childbirth yantra in the classic labyrinth form with opening at the top from Rjasthan or Gujarat, dating ca 1750. The writing on the original manuscript in Hindi (not shown here) describes the ritual, still practiced today in northwest India, of drawing the labyrinth in saffron on a metal plate, rinsing the plate and drinking the water to alleviate labor pains.[8]

To fully appreciate this yantra, make a drawing or painting of one, then meditate on it using your eyes to move down through it.

THE SEVEN FOLDS OF THIS LABYRINTH represent the mythical seven chambers of the mother's womb,* leading down and out the birth canal. Written in Hindi below this drawing was a description of drawing and drinking the saffron labyrinth in childbirth.

Three sacred mantras are written in Hindi below the horizontal line, from left to right: Om, shrim and hrim.[9]

OM: Many mantras begin and end with om. om is the mantra of assent; it means yes and affirms and energizes whatever we say after it. It also gives strength, protection and grace.

SHRIM: (Pronounced Shreem) is a mantra of love, devotion and beauty. It takes us to the heart and gives faith and steadiness to our emotional nature, allowing us to surrender to, or be immersed in, whatever we offer the mantra to.

HRIM: (Pronounced Hreem) awakens us at a soul or heart level, connecting us to Divine forces of love and attraction.[10]

*In a pen and ink drawing, Leonardo da Vinci made an anatomical cross-section study expressing the medieval idea the the hollow interior of the uterus is divided into seven cells. [11]

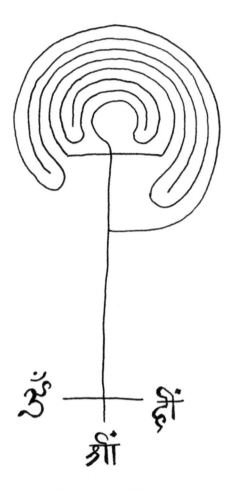

ABHYUMAN YANTRA

This childbirth yantra was drawn with pen and red ink on paper during the nineteenth-century in Rajasthan.[12]

Chakra-Vyūha

IN SANSKRIT, 'CHAKRA' MEANS "WHEEL", and "Vyūha" refers to an ancient battle formation. This labyrinth represents the impenetrable defense formation used by armed soldiers and described in the epic Indian poem, *Mahabharata*. The battle was between the Pandavas and Kauravas. After ten days in battle, although many died trying, the Pandavas could not penetrate the labyrinthine battle formation held by the Kauravas. A young warrior and Pandava hero, Abhmanyu, was summoned because he knew how to penetrate the battle formation. How did this warrior know the secret?

When he was in his mother's womb, his father Arjuna told his mother about this magical labyrinthine formation. She listened attentively to the part about how to enter the labyrinth, how soldiers could battle their way to the center, but then she fell asleep. She did not hear—and therefore Abhmanyu did not hear—how a soldier could successfully fight his way out of the labyrinthine formation.

Abhmanyu successfuly penetrated the Chakra-Vyūha labyrinth, fighting his way to the center. Victory was in reach for the Abhmanyu and the Pandavas. But in the center Abhmanyu was killed in a shower of arrows. Perhaps this is a story about incomplete initiation.[13]

The Chakra-Vyūha labyrinth was, and still is, used as a talisman in birth. I like to think of this labyrinth as the Warrior's labyrinth, and that tracing it ensures the mother's victory in her battle with fear, pain, and the unknown in labor. [14]

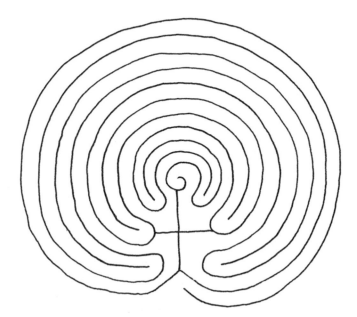

CHAKRA-VYŪHA OR PADMAVŪHA

This eleven-circuit labyrinth was found in a modern book of Indian rituals. The text reads:

> *"Rub ocher [saffron?] with water from the Ganges and use it to draw the chakra-vyūh on a bronze plate, rinse it off with water from the Ganges, then give it to the laboring mother to drink and birth will shortly ensue and the pain of labor will be eased. Coupled with the healing properties of the Ganges, this saffron water is thought to retain the powers of the dissolved labyrinth drawing."[15]*

Gewant Yantra

THIS CHILDBIRTH YANTRA WAS MADE BY MAVIS GEWANT, a sacred artist, childbirth educator, doula and mother; she used this yantra with the births of her two sons.

The yantra design represents the microcosm of the macrocosm. Every shape and form emits a specific form or vibration, as follows:

The square (*bhupur*) represents the earth element (*prihivi*) and is the seat or base of the yantra. Within the square are the eight directions; beginning at the top, which represents east, then moving clockwise. The four "gates" (the protrusions on the square) allow the energy or breath to move in and out of the yantra.

The circle (*chakra*) represents evolution, rotation as with the spiral; it is associated with perfection and the blissful creative void.

The eight petals represent the lotus (*padma*), and symbolize purity. The yantra lotus signifies freedom from interference with the outside, a symbol of the absolute force or Supreme Self.[16] Eight petals may also represent the five elements: earth, water, fire, air, ether (*akash*), and the three *gunas*: light or pure energy, fiery or very active energy and inertia.

The lotus petals and the circles create movement and flow, symbols of opening.

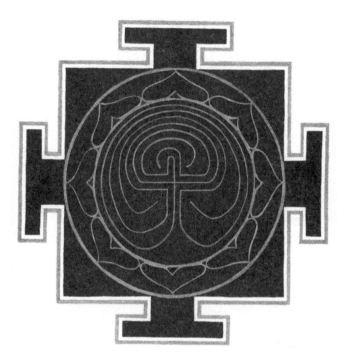

CHILDBIRTH YANTRA BY MAVIS GEWANT

Nazca Animal Labyrinths

Peru's animal labyrinths are one-of-a-kind and mysterious in many ways. In the 1920s, the first pilots to fly over Peru noticed hundreds of geometric shapes, including about 70 animal figures, "drawn" in the flat, parched southwestern corner of Peru, north of the small town of Nazca, between the coast and the Andes. These labyrinths are so large, their shapes can only be seen and understood from local hillsides and from the air; the largest is 285 feet long.

The animal and geometric shaped labyrinths were made over an extended period of time, possibly beginning 2000 years ago.[17] Nobody knows why the ancients made these labyrinths on such a large scale, perhaps they were for ceremonial walking or processions, or perhaps they imagined that their ancestors or the Holy Spirit could see the images from above. Even though we don't know if the ancients used the animal labyrinths for childbirth meditation, I included them in this section because many women find it helpful to identify with animals that birth easily, are good or fiercely-protective mothers, or have other qualities they want to embody or develop as they become mothers themselves.

The Nazca labyrinths consist of a single line that "traces" the shape of the animal. Where the line begins marks the entrance, the line that outlines the shape is the pathway, and the exit marks where the line ends. Instead of walking the path between the lines (as is typical with most other labyrinths), one walks on, or finger traces on, the line.

Many of the animals portrayed in the labyrinths at Nazca are not native to the area, including the spider and the monkey shown here. A hummingbird, lizard, shark, whale, pelican, and dog are among the animals represented at Nazca. The drawings shown here of the Spider and Monkey labyrinths replicate aerial photos.

The Spider Labyrinth *is modeled after a rare, tiny spider found only found in the most remote parts of the Amazon jungle. These spiders are only five to ten millimeters in length, but the Nazca Spider labyrinth is 45 yards long, and its jaw is eight feet. In the 1950s, using a microscope, it was discovered that this Amazon spider carries her eggs only on her second to last leg on the right.*[18] *What's really amazing is that the second to the last leg on the right on the labyrinth Spider is visibly longer and is the entrance to the labyrinth.*

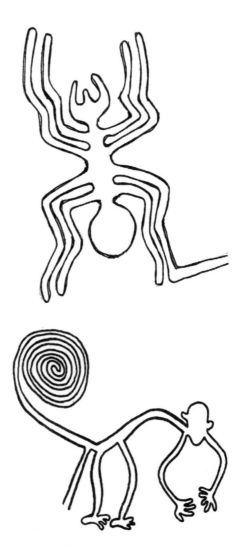

The Nazca Monkey *is over 80 yards long, a little less than the length of a football field! The entrance to the monkey is at its root chakra, or rectum. Nazca labyrinths had "mirror" paths, which means you walk on, or finger-trace on, the line, not between the lines. To begin, follow one of the root chakra lines up (right or left), and trace the monkey.*

I have shown you a sampling of labyrinths found all over the world. Now it is time to learn how the labyrinth is relevant to you as you prepare for labor, how labor is like a labyrinth, and how to make your own *Laborinth*, a modern meditation labyrinth for your labor.

Labor is a Labyrinth

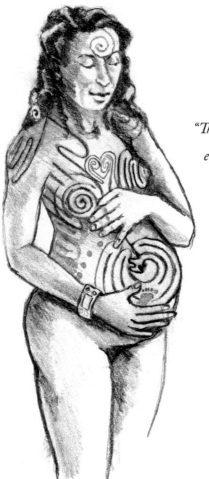

*"The first path a human being
ever travels
is the path that leads
out of the maternal womb.
Every human being's first labyrinth
is that of woman."*

—Jacques Attali,
The Labyrinth in Culture and Society

Labor is a Labyrinth

ONCE YOU ENTER A LABYRINTH, the continuous, winding, twisting-and-turning pathway eventually leads you to the center and out again. The same thing happens once your water breaks or contractions begin; there is nothing you need to plan in order to walk, one contraction at a time, to the center where you meet your baby, and then find your way out of the postpartum labyrinth.

Hairpin turns in the labyrinth disorient your sense of direction, inducing doubt and confusion. Unpredictable, sudden changes in direction in the labyrinth parallel unexpected, unwished-for surprises that are part of every labor and postpartum.

As the pathways wind back and forth toward the center of the labyrinth, you may begin thinking that you are back where you started, or that you are getting nowhere, or that you are moving away from your "goal." The same thing often happens during labor. From time to time, like most mothers, you will feel "lost" in labor because when you are *in* labor, you can't see how far you've come, or how close you are to giving birth.

> *When the road goes straight, I romp ahead;*
> *when it twists and turns, I make the best of it I can.*
> —Lieh-tzû, *Taoist Master*[1]

THE LABYRINTH CAN ALSO REPRESENT THE HERO'S JOURNEY, which has three phases: Preparation, Ordeal, and Return. Although the Ordeal can be lived during conception, pregnancy, labor, or postpartum, to keep things simple for this book, I will refer to pregnancy as the Preparation phase, labor as the Ordeal, and postpartum as the Return.

Preparation takes place before you cross the Threshold and enter your Laborinth. There are two phases of Preparation, one unconscious and the other conscious, or intentional. The unconscious phase of preparation begins long before you are pregnant; it begins in childhood and includes all of your cultural conditioning and life experiences. In contrast, acts of intentional preparation include taking childbirth classes, reading, and "eating for two."

A labyrinth's path is only wide open from the mouth to the center and out again *on paper*! It's rarely that simple in life or in labor, even when the birth is "normal." The journey from the mouth of your Laborinth to the center represents the **Ordeal** phase of the hero's journey. As a hero-mother, during labor you enter the unknown, face your Tiger* or Dragon, and undergo a psychic and social transformation which includes the inevitable death of ego, expectations and old beliefs.

During a rite of passage, an initiate passes through seven Thresholds or Gates. If these Gates had names, they might be called the Gates of Great Doubt, Great Faith, Great Love, Great Determination, Mother Intuition, Mercy, Holy Terror, and Deep Surrender, to name just a few. Since birth is a rite of passage, you should expect to pass through at least a few emotional, mental, and/or psychic Gates during your childbearing year, although you cannot anticipate or choose how they will manifest for you.

Before you reach the Center, or Womb, of your Laborinth—which represents the birth of your child and your birth as a mother—you will come *(even in normal labor)* to a Gate of Great Doubt. At this Gate you may doubt many things, including: your ability to cope, your intuition, or even that labor will ever end. It has been said that you can't really experience Great Trust or Faith unless you've passed through the Gate of Great Doubt. Even if you are consumed with doubt, reaching the Center of your Laborinth or labor is inevitable if you just keep stepping forward, one step and one breath at a time.

Tiger represents our imagined fears. The Tiger either stalks us and we freeze in fear, or we stalk the Tiger and thus become more resourceful and able to cope. See Birthing From Within, pages 118-120.

After learning about the Laborinth a home-birth assistant said,
"Most of the women I work with don't experience those twists and turns because they
birth normally".

On the contrary!

The Laborinth is not a symbol for complicated or medicalized labor.
It is a symbol of a woman's inner experience of labor (and life!).

There is an expectation or ideal that women should "trust labor," with the implication that if they trust their bodies and the process enough, they will be calm and labor will be normal. I suggest that this idea of Trust be expanded to include trusting even crazy thoughts and emotions which come and go during labor and postpartum, because this is a normal response to being in the Unknown. Trust that you *will* be surprised at least once in your Ordeal. Trust that you will experience a range of feelings and strategies as you make your way through labor and your Laborinth: confidence, doubt, fear, fierce determination, trust, wanting to give up, wanting to be in control. Trust that losing your innocence and trust is part *of* the process rather than an interference *in* the process.

Instead of trying to avoid surprises, look for the Gate of Not-Knowing. Look for the Gate of the Unexpected. That way, when you come to it, since you expected it, you may only feel half as surprised or lost.

Just when you think you've hit a wall in labor, you will turn a corner and the path will lead you in a new direction. The Labyrinth symbol reminds us that we can't predict or plan the absolute course of life or labor.

During an Ordeal, the mind always looks for shortcuts. In a labyrinth there are no shortcuts; if you try to cross lines to get "there" faster, you will not know which way to turn next. Remember: in a labyrinth, and in labor, there's nothing to figure out. You don't need to "get it right" to earn love or respect or to be a good-enough mother. When you realize this, you will pass through the Gate of Great Love.

The labyrinth brings thought patterns and strategies
to conscious awareness, and so does labor.

Do your best, as you know it in each moment. Love yourself, especially when you are lost. Even when you don't know what to do, take one small step. *Know* that your baby will be born and labor will end.

The **Center** represents the place of endings and beginnings. It is the place where labor ends, where your life as you knew it "ends." It is the place where your baby is born, where you are born as a mother.

After reaching the center, after giving birth, the journey is not yet over. Although you will rest and "cocoon" in the center with your newly born baby a while, you cannot stay in the center. When the time comes, you will begin the **Return** phase of your journey, i.e., your transition to parenthood (which often feels like another Ordeal!).

Turn around in the center of your Laborinth and continue taking one step at a time. The medical model defines postpartum as a six-week period, but studies show it takes parents three years to make the psychological and social Return. Regardless of messages from society, you cannot "cross lines" to get out quickly.

Eventually, and it may take the three years, you will come to the final Threshold, and step out of your Laborinth.

The Return

THE RETURN IS A VITALLY IMPORTANT PART OF THE HEROINE'S JOURNEY; it cannot be rushed. Do not expect to give birth, turn around, step into your old footsteps and walk back into your old life. Birth changes everything. You not only gave birth to a child and you gave birth to yourself as a Mother (or Father). For that transformation to have occurred, you had to have been stripped of certain ideas or ideals. Perhaps the Ordeal tested and even ravaged your body. The person you were when you begin this journey is not the same "you" who will return. You will return in your new identity as a mother. During your Return, everything changes, even your body changes; not even your old wardrobe and shoes fit.

While you were in labor and cocooning postpartum with your baby, the world went on without you. During your Return, what you are thinking about and what you have to say may seem out of sync with most people, especially friends who aren't parents or who haven't made the journey that you have made.

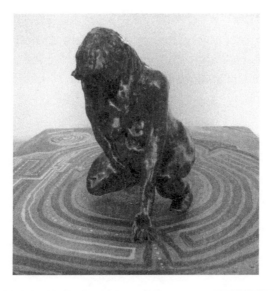

Birth changes everything. You and your partner won't and can't return to your relationship as it was before. When using the labyrinth tool, it generally takes as much time to exit the labyrinth as it took to enter. However, in life and in your living-Laborinth, it may take two or three years to completely "exit." It often takes that long to fully integrate your birth experience and your transformation into being a parent. Laborinth meditations and rituals can help you contemplate and integrate your birth story and your Return (see pages 61-102).

When you first leave the center of your Laborinth, the pathways wrap around and are close to the center; this parallels your immediate postpartum experience. For weeks and months after giving birth, you will be thinking about what happened in labor and wanting to tell or write all the important details of your story. Visitors will come to see you and the baby. At first they will want to hear your birth story, bring you food and presents and give you advice. But after a while, like the pathways, your old friends, even your family or partner, may seem far away. Frequent feedings or struggles with breastfeeding can be all-consuming. The long stretches in the labyrinth's pathways might parallel long, sleepless nights, feelings of isolation from friends, work, and your former life and routines.

There are no shortcuts on the Return. It takes time to retrace the labyrinthine path. It takes even longer while carrying and caring for your baby. The non-linear, convoluted, and unpredictable twists and turns in the labyrinth aptly represent your transition to parenthood.

How to Make Your *Laborinth*

Now that you've learned about "labyrinths" as a tool for meditation and childbirth, you might like to make your own labyrinth, or Laborinth, to hold in your hand or hang on the wall in your labor room and to use as a tool for meditation. Our Laborinth is different from other labyrinths because it includes a symbolic Threshold, Footprints and the artists' personal symbols. The Laborinth was my invention for my childbirth classes and doesn't exist in other cultures. First, I want you to show you a few Laborinths so you can appreciate the variety.

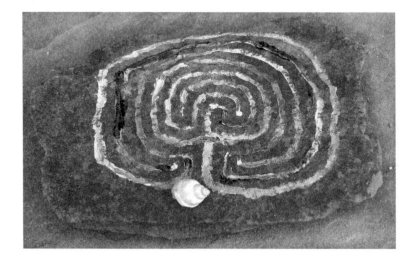

I painted my Laborinth on a rock because I want to be Ginger's "rock" in labor. I put a shell we found at the beach on our honeymoon for the Threshold. We learned that the left-handed labyrinth is masculine, so I made mine this way.

— A father

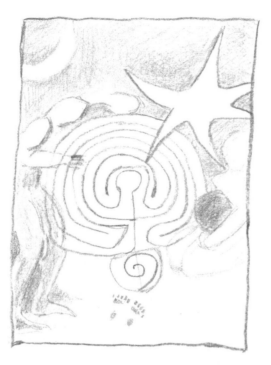

I am thankful for the Laborinth and the time spent drawing and exploring what it represents to me. With the birth of my first child, we had a lovely home birth planned, but things didn't exactly go as planned. Keeping the idea of the labyrinth in my head helped me to deal with every twist and turn that confronted us as labor progressed. I was faced with nurses, doctors and stark white light in my face as opposed to the intimate candlelit birth we had planned. Our second baby is due in a month; we are planning a home birth. I am focused on the Center and am not afraid of the twists and turns that the Laborinth will inevitably take. I trust myself and know that in whatever direction the Laborinth may take me, it will lead me in the right direction.

— A mother

How to Create Your Laborinth

For many years, Parents in my Birthing From Within classes learned how the childbearing year is like a labyrinth, and how to draw a seven -circuit labyrinth. Making and meditating on their own Laborinth is among the most favored activities. First-time parents resonate with the Laborinth. Parents experienced in birth unanimously agree that the inner experience of labor and postpartum is just like traveling through a labyrinth.

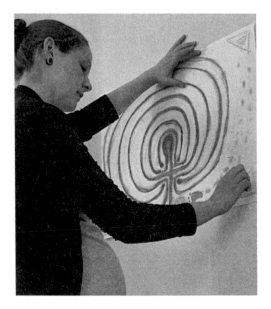

You have been learning how childbirth labyrinths have been a tradition around the world and about a variety of labyrinth meditations and ceremonies. Now it is time for you to make your own Laborinth. First, you will learn how to draw a classic seven-circuit labyrinth. In the pages that follow, you will learn the meaning of Footprints and Threshold, and add these symbols to your drawing.

What you will need:

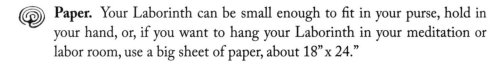 **The "seed."** Every labyrinth begins with a "seed:" a simple pattern from which the rest of the labyrinth grows. The seed shown here is for the classic seven-circuit labyrinth. There are more seeds for different labyrinth designs in the Appendix at the end of this book.

Paper. Your Laborinth can be small enough to fit in your purse, hold in your hand, or, if you want to hang your Laborinth in your meditation or labor room, use a big sheet of paper, about 18" x 24."

Soft art pastels. Perfect for making a big labyrinth (avoid using magic markers, crayons, oil pastels or the waxy, hard pastels sold in office supply stores). Pastels are "forgiving;" if a mistake is made, simply rub out or blend in the mistake.

Paint. Once you learn to draw labyrinths, you may want to paint your Laborinth or yantra using tempera, acrylic or watercolors on thick watercolor paper or canvas.

Fixative. When your Laborinth is complete, hair spray or special pastel fixative will preserve your drawing and keep the colors from smudging or rubbing off.

This Seed has been passed

from person to person,

from midwife to mother,

from mother to daughter,

from one culture to another,

for four thousand years.

Now it is being passed to you.

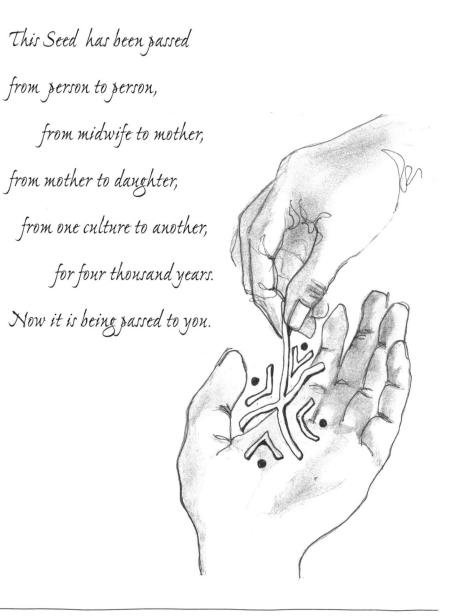

Step One: Draw a Labyrinth

C HOOSE ANY TWO COLORS OF PASTELS. Use one color to draw the "seed" and the other to draw the pathway lines. Using two colors allows you to always see the seed pattern, which makes it easier to know where to connect each corridor to the "seed." If a mistake is made, with two colors it's easier to see where it was made, so it can be easily corrected. Later, if you like, you can blend the colors together. Once you become experienced in drawing labyrinths, you might only use one color for the seed and the pathways.

Labyrinths grow upwards and outwards as you draw them, so you need to draw your "seed" about one-third up from the bottom of the paper, and centered from right to left.

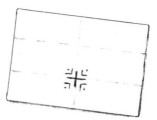

Next, draw the corridors. Begin by drawing an arch from the vertical center line (in the +) to the first vertical line of the "picture frame corner" on the left. Follow the illustrations on the next page. Continue connecting the next line or dot on the right with the next line or dot on the left.

When drawing your paths, you can make the corners square or round. Make an effort to draw the width of the pathways consistently throughout, and at least as wide as your finger so you can trace the path.

RIGHT-HANDED AND LEFT-HANDED LABYRINTHS

Labyrinths are referred to as right-handed or left-handed which refers to the direction of the first turn after you enter the labyrinth. If it is a right-handed turn, it is associated with Mother Earth and the Great-Feminine. The left-handed labyrinth is associated with the Sun and Divine-Masculine.

To make the "Feminine" labyrinth, the first line you draw from the center goes left. To make a "Masculine" labyrinth, draw the first line that forms the center to the right.[1]

DRAWING THE PATHWAYS STEP-BY-STEP

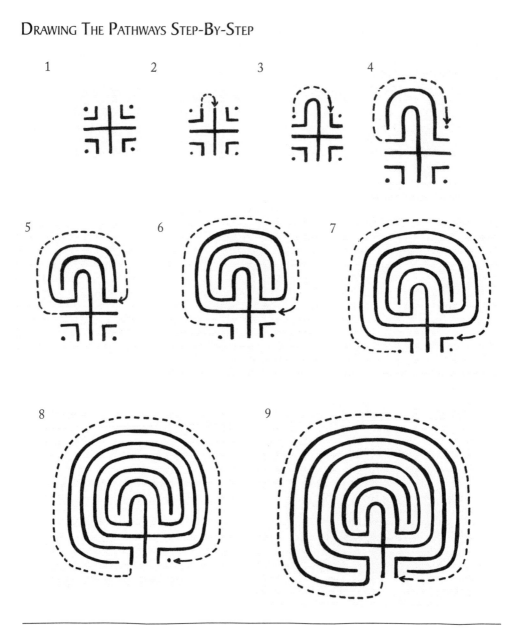

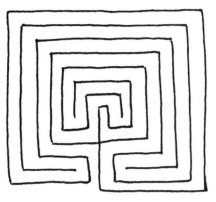

When drawing your paths, you can make the corners square or round.
Remember to draw the width of the pathways at least as wide as your finger
so you can trace the path.

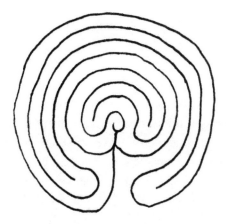

Step Two: Draw Your Footprints

After you draw your Laborinth,

draw your footprints about two inches before the entrance

to represent the ground of your knowing and freedom.

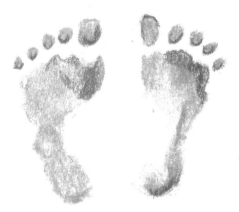

Footprints are a symbol for everything you have lived, for every step you have taken through life that brought you here to this moment. Footprints before the mouth of your Laborinth represent your conscious and unconscious assumptions, beliefs and expectations. You cannot fully know them, or their significance, before you make the journey. Finally, your Footprints serve to remind you that you cannot "think" your way through labor. You must act, move, keep moving—even when you aren't certain where you are or where the next step leads.

In preparation for most journeys, you dress up and
   put on comfortable shoes or hiking boots
      to protect your feet and to help you make ground quickly.

For journeys of the Heart, for labyrinthine journeys into the
   unknown, the underworld, or Laborland,
      you cannot rush toward your imagined goal.
So, begin your journey
   by symbolically taking off your comfortable shoes or
      muddy boots.

Walk barefoot through life and labor
feeling each step
of your way.

Stand open and quietly resolute before entering your Laborinth.
   Draw energy from Mother Earth.

Face what lies before you as the Birth Warrior
   you are becoming. Close your eyes, and...

STEP INTO THE MYSTERY OF BIRTH.

Step Three: Draw Your Threshold

After you draw your Footprints, draw a Threshold.

Make it wide enough to completely cover the opening to your Laborinth,

and high or awesome enough that you would have to pause before it

(not simply walk around it or over it), before entering your Laborinth.

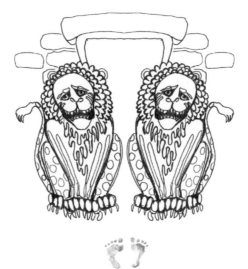

THRESHOLDS ARE UNIVERSAL, ARCHITECTURAL SYMBOLS of transition and transcendence. They also represent the separation of two worlds: the known and the unknown, the mundane and the sacred. In birth, the Threshold separates the worlds of Maidens and of Mothers. Standing before a threshold, you stand in the liminal, in-between place. You are between conditioned-knowing and soul-knowing. You are between clinging to the security of known comforts and stepping onto the swinging bridge over a chasm of fire that leads you to self-love.

Before the small portal to the Neolithic tomb at New Grange in Ireland is an awesome mega-ton threshold stone ornately carved with spirals, diamonds and waves. When I first stood before it, I sensed, by its imposing size, that this threshold was purposeful—it would have made the Neolithic people pause before entering the tomb. We too must pause between leaving our ordinary world and entering sacred space or our birth space, and again when leaving ceremonial space before re-entering the mundane world.

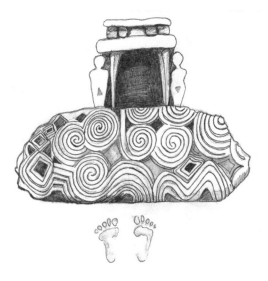

Stand before your Threshold.
Remember your deepest question or intention,
forget everything you think you know or planned.
Send a prayer of gratitude.
Call on your ancestors, angels or allies.

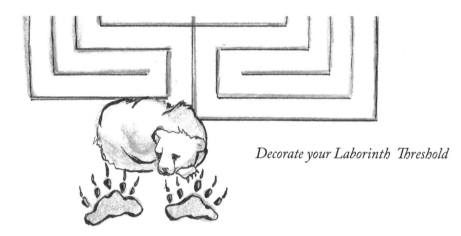

Decorate your Laborinth Threshold

DECORATE YOUR THRESHOLD with symbols or words that hold personal meaning for you. There are as many artistic expressions of the Threshold as there are symbolic meanings for it. Your Threshold could be a simple line, or a lion; it could be a sprinkling of rose petals or a gate. Sometimes I draw a butterfly for transformation, or a heart with a hole in it to represent crossing with an open heart. This Bear threshold is a reminder that entering the unknown is like entering the long solitude of the winter cave. Hibernation may represent accessing our unconscious or deep Feminine and giving birth to new personal power. On the way out of the labyrinth or Ordeal, we cross the springtime threshold with new instincts.

Completely covering the opening to your Laborinth with a substantial Threshold could be a symbolic representation for putting a tight lid on the proverbial "cooking pot" of labor and life and not allowing heat or flavor to escape before you are fully cooked. This brings to mind Rumi's chickpea poem:

A chickpea leaps almost over the rim of the pot
where it is being boiled.
'Why are you doing this to me?'
The cook knocks him down with the ladle.
'Don't you try to jump out.
You think I'm torturing you.
I'm giving you flavor.
So you can mix with spices and rice.'

Now that you've completed drawing your Laborinth, complete with Footprints and Threshold, you're ready to try out your new labyrinth!

As you use your Laborinth, the pastel pathways will smear, blend and soften. Check to make sure the pathway is continuous from the mouth to the center. If it's not, correct it by going back to the original seed lines and retrace your steps until you find the error. "Erase" the error in the pastel pathway by buffing and blending it into the pathway, then draw the new lines.

Before you enter, take a moment to settle. Decide which meditation practice (pages 61-102) you will use while tracing your Laborinth.

Begin finger-tracing the path with your non-dominant hand. This will help you access intuition and stay open to feelings, memories, and images. Go all the way to the center and out again. Consider tracing your labyrinth by candlelight, three to seven times consecutively to further quiet your mind and deepen your meditation.

Pause anytime to be with what comes up, but don't stop completely, or quit, in the middle of the labyrinth. Continue, even going slowly, all the way to the center, and out again.

In the Center, connect with your own Center. Throughout, be receptive.

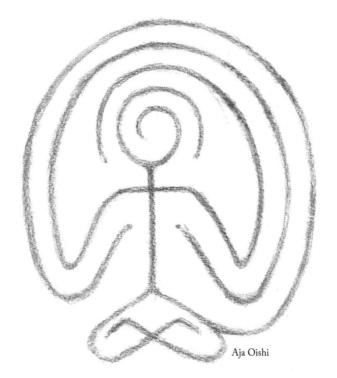

Aja Oishi

Meditations

and

Ceremonies

How to Enter a Labyrinth Meditation

Your first step into the labyrinth is an inward one.

THE LABYRINTH PATH AND MEDITATIONS parallel the hero's JOURNEY. The hero does not rush into her Ordeal or initiation, she prepares for it. So take as much time as you need to prepare for your labyrinth walk and meditations. We tend to live too-full lives, rushing from one thing to another. You can walk or trace a labyrinth in five to fifteen minutes, cross it off your list—then hurry on to the next thing in your day, but this approach won't serve you. Plan on spending fifteen minutes to an hour, to give yourself time to settle before entering to fully experience the labyrinth as meditation.

It is very important to pause or meditate before entering the labyrinth. During this interlude, you begin to leave the turmoil and noise of the world behind. Decide how you will dedicate this labyrinth walk or meditation. Although you may start with an intention, allow for something new to enter your mind as you make your way through and out of the labyrinth.

Before entering, consider that you are not making this journey alone; you are following in the footsteps of your parents, mentors, ancestors, and all women through time and space who have come this way before you. Invite allies, angels, and ancestors to accompany and assist you through the labyrinth, labor, and life. You might even ask their permission to enter.

Before entering or leaving the labyrinth, theologian Thomas Moore suggests a "body prayer."[1] A body prayer is a silent gesture, such as raising your hands above your head to receive the sun or moon's rays, or reaching out as if to embrace the whole earth and all sentient beings, or bowing to embody your intention to become empty and receptive.

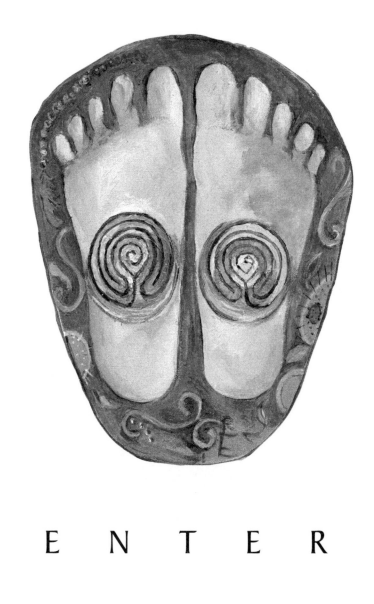

E N T E R

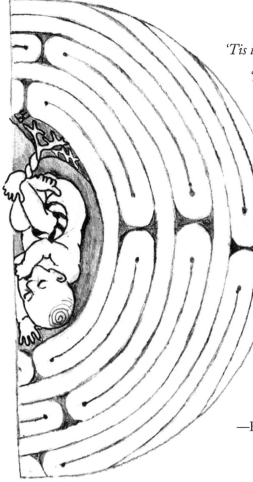

'Tis the gift to be simple,
   'tis the gift to be free,
     'Tis the gift to come down
      where we ought to be,
       And when we find ourselves
        in the place just right,
         'Twill be in the valley of
         love and delight.
          When true simplicity is gain'd,
         To bow and to bend
         we shan't be asham'd,
       To turn, turn will be our delight,
     Till by turning, turning
   we come 'round right.

—Elder Joseph Bracken. Jr.

Sacred Pathway

Preparing for the center is something that you do at each step along the pathway... Each moment of attention to your walk, to your physical body, and emotions slowly quiets your mental chatter; each repetition of the meditation serves to take you deeper into your inner world... moving away from your past into the future. There is often a sense of making yourself ready for that which is to come.

—Helen Curry, *The Way of the Labyrinth*

LABYRINTHINE PATHWAYS REPRESENT LIFE and meandering through life. When entering a seven-circuit labyrinth, it seems the perceived "goal" (the center) is within reach just beyond the first wall; this is analogous to some mothers' initial optimism or excitement when labor begins.

Soon after entering the labyrinth, you encounter a turn, and then another. Each turn appears to take you further away from the center, your "goal," or intention, which will remain out of sight for a while. Sometimes the path is wide open and progress seems effortless. The unpredictable twists and turns and ups and downs in the labyrinth might be analogous to your mind, emotions, actual events in labor, or a change of heart when you meet unexpected and unwished-for surprises. There is no turning back; there are no short-cuts or detours to avoid what lies in the path. Simply keep moving forward by putting one foot in front of the other until you reach the center.

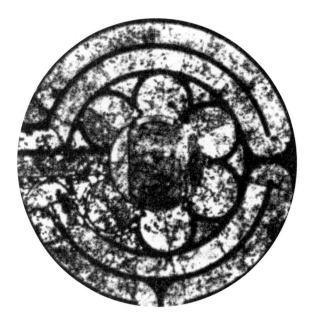

CENTER ROSETTE

The center of labyrinth in Chartres Cathedral, France

"The symbol of the Center is the blue rose, the golden flower ... the meeting and conjunction of the conscious and unconscious... if the lover and the beloved."[2] The Center at Chartres is a six-petal rosette associated with the Rose of Sharon (a normal rose has five petals). In the Middle Ages, the rose was a symbol for the Virgin Mary, of human and divine love, of passionate love, and of a love beyond passion. A single rose represented God's love for the world. Six petals were associated with the sixth day of creation, trial, effort, and cessation of movement after God created man. The number six represents the human soul, six directions of space, harmony, balance, sincerity, calm unfolding, and forgiveness.

In the Center of the Labyrinth

Earth Mother
birthing instrument.
Birth and rebirth.
In labyrinth rituals across cultures
women were literally at the Center.
—Helen Curry, *The Way of the Labyrinth*

EVERY INHABITED PLACE, even your own home, has one or more centers. The Center is the heart or soul of that place. In every Great Story there is a sacred Center, the place where the heavens and earth intersect. This Center was often a Holy Mountain, a Cosmic Tree, or the carefully chosen place on which ziggurats, temples, churches, or altars were built. Emergence myths describe the Center of the World as the navel of the earth from where humans were "born."

In the labyrinth of birth, the winding pathways represent pregnancy, labor, and postpartum. The open Center represents the womb and the "birth" of the baby, mother, and father. In medieval times, it represented the Virgin Mary.

As an ancient instrument for meditation and healing, use the labyrinth to practice moving from and being in your Center each "step" of the way. Students of martial arts learn that the physical center of the body, also called the "seat" of power, is two inches below the navel. It is where "your physical body was first knitted together after conception in your mother's womb."[3] To strengthen the feeling of being centered, focus your attention on your center as you move through the labyrinth. You can continue this practice in your everyday life, e.g., while walking, cooking, and bathing.

WHAT TO DO IN THE CENTER OF A LABYRINTH

Turn by turn, from the mouth of the labyrinth to the center, worries, grief, body tension, and mind chatter fall away. As we approach the open, empty space of the labyrinth's center, we are in a more receptive state of mind. When we reach the center, we often feel a spontaneous shift in our emotions; even our initial intention may transform or disappear altogether. It is here, in the center, after making tremendous effort, that, when we stop and do nothing, we often receive an epiphany, an answer to our deepest question, or a solution to a problem. The open, empty place in the Center contains infinite possibilities; you may see or hear what you have not yet realized.

If you are finger-tracing or scanning the labyrinth with your eyes, when you arrive in the center, close your eyes. Notice any images or insights that come spontaneously. If you are walking a labyrinth, and space and time allow, take a few minutes to sit quietly in the center. Do not sit there thinking, problem-solving, or journaling. Do nothing: be quiet and listen within. Your journey is not yet complete. Turn around, and while staying in your Center, begin making your exit. Retracing your steps helps you to integrate the gift you received into your body and mind—so you can bring it to the world.

PLEASE, DON'T BE A LABYRINTH LITTERBUG

One evening, in preparation for leading a labyrinth workshop the following day, I walked the labyrinth myself. Upon reaching the center, I was instantly pulled out of my own experience when distracted by weathered clutter left by others on the rocks, tucked in between the rocks, and piled up in the center. The variety of tokens included money, beads, talismans, paper tied in ribbons, stuffed animals, rocks with words written on them, and whatnot. In a breath, my attention shifted from inward to outward.

To leave tokens in the Center defies the essence of labyrinth meditation, which is to allow yourself (and others) to be utterly receptive. If you are inclined to bring something and leave it behind, inquire within about what magical thinking is leading you to leave a token in the center of a labyrinth, especially a public one. For whom are you leaving it? Please, don't litter in the labyrinth.

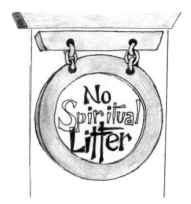

How to Exit Your Labyrinth

Since the entrance has now become the exit,
let this be a reminder that all endings are beginnings
and all beginnings are endings.
—London and Recio, *Sacred Rituals*

LEAVING THE LABYRINTH parallels your postpartum "Return." It is a vitally important part of the heroine's journey; it cannot be rushed. With each step, you are leaving something old behind, and integrating something new in your whole being. With each step, make a conscious effort to be centered and in the moment.

In the same way that getting to the center of the labyrinth is not the goal when entering the labyrinth, getting out of the labyrinth is not the goal during the journey out. During your "Return," or exit, make an effort to gradually integrate insights or shifts you may have had, while still being receptive to new ones that occur in this phase.

Approaching the mouth of the labyrinth, you will anticipate or see the Threshold from the other side. It might bring up the same feelings and patterns of thought you experience when you anticipate the end of any journey, whether it is vacation, a relationship, or labor. What do you do or tell yourself as you approach the "finish line?" Do you feel tired? Do you begin to rush to get to the end, and get back to your life, forgetting your intention or mantra? The labyrinth is a mirror that shows you how you live, think, and strategize. You may discover that who you are inside and outside the labyrinth are the same. Do you linger, delaying the inevitable, trying to hold on to the special experience you just had?

You will eventually cross the Threshold and return to "your life." When your integration is complete, you bring new knowledge into your life that will serve you and everyone you touch.

Breath Awareness in the Labyrinth

Wherever you go, you still have to breathe.
—Seiju, Abbot of Albuquerque Zen Center

B REATHING IN THE LABYRINTH, in life, form a continuum in your life. You can practice Breath Awareness meditation in the labyrinth during pregnancy, labor, and postpartum.

Breathing is involuntary. Your body knows how quickly, slowly, or deeply to breathe in response to levels of carbon dioxide and activity. Unless you have a respiratory problem, you trust your body to breathe on its own. So, during meditation or labor, don't conjure up special breath patterns. Trust your body; trust your breath. Simply witness the perfection of your body's breathing on its own. Pay particular attention to the exhalation, the breath of letting go and release.

Just when the mind begins to unwind and let go in labor or in the labyrinth, you may start thinking, looking for a way out, or spinning strategies to avoid one thing or achieve another. It is this kind of thinking that causes suffering. You might eventually find a way out of a predicament. Labor always comes to an end. But the suffering that comes from "monkey mind" goes on unless your attention is focused on a single point. Your outward breath can be that focal point.

The mind only generates one thought at a time, and usually it is not thinking about breathing. At the same time, your body is breathing on its own (whether you think about it or not). When you commit to being *completely focused* on your next outward breath as you move through the labyrinth, you may gradually enter a more meditative state of mind.

Labyrinth as a Tool for Prenatal Pain-Coping Practice

To deepen your mastery of Breath Awareness in preparation for coping with pain in labor, hold an ice cube in one hand, while walking or finger-tracing the labyrinth with the other. It's easy to trace a labyrinth or meditate when you are comfortable. Holding an ice cube or putting a hand in a bowl of ice water while tracing the labyrinth (with your eyes or the other hand) requires more concentration. By adding "ice-contractions" to your prenatal meditation, you are training your mind to concentrate in labor. Then, like the women in northwest India who trace the childbirth yantra with their eyes while in labor, you will benefit even more from the labyrinth as a tool for working with the intensity of labor.

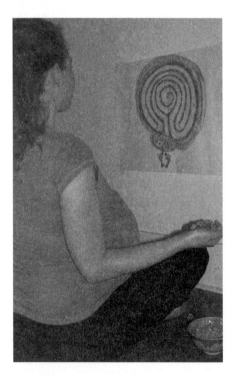

Instructions for Breath Awareness

Before entering the labyrinth (and a contraction):

- Bring your full attention to your breathing.

- Notice exactly when your exhalation begins—and ends.

- Make no effort to change your breathing in any way. Breath Awareness is rooted in a trust that the body breathes on its own *perfectly* in the labyrinth, in life, and in labor.

In the pathways:

- Walk through, or glide your finger along, the corridor in unison with your outward breath, as if your exhalation is propelling you through the corridor. As you breathe in, you may pause or slow down. There are no absolute rules here; do whatever comes naturally.

- If your mind begins to think, wander, or look for a way out—don't think or judge yourself for thinking! Simply bring your attention back to your next outward breath. Immerse your whole being in your next outward breath and your next step forward, and keep going.

(For more instruction on Breath Awareness and other pain-coping practices, read *Ancient Map for Modern Birth* and listen to my five free audio-recordings teaching *Pain-Coping Practices for Parents* on sevengatesmedia.com.)

Contemplate Your Heart's Burning Question

Knowing your personal question is central to birth preparation.
Whatever your question is, leave no stone unturned.
Ask your question often and look at it from every angle until your conscious
mind is exhausted, and your heart is receptive to answers.

WHAT IS IT YOU REALLY WANT TO KNOW, OR TO BEGIN LIVING, NOW? Before entering the labyrinth, take time to formulate your Heart's Question. Try to keep it short and straightforward. A good place to begin preparing for birth or parenting is with your heart's burning question. For example:

- How am I bringing true love to this moment?" (Then do it!)

- What does this moment need? (Then do it!)

- "At what chasm's edge am I at this moment?" —Mircea Eliade[4]

Keeping your question short allows you to ask it silently with every exhalation, and to be receptive to, or "listen" for, the answer with every in-breath. Or, you might ask the first half of your question on your in-breath and the second half on the out-breath.

However you pace yourself, commit yourself to walking from the entrance to the center while immersed in your Heart's Question. Don't think about solutions or answers or try to come up with the answer yourself. Simply ask your Question and keep walking. Breathe and listen steadily. Be patient. Sometimes answers come after you stop trying to figure it out, or after you've exited the labyrinth.

If you finish walking the labyrinth and realize you never got out of your head, you may want to walk or trace the labyrinth again, more slowly and mindfully, to get into a meditative state of mind. Some people trace the seven-circuit labyrinth seven times to achieve deeper meditation.

Here's a tip: If your Question could be answered with a "yes" or "no," or with logical information from a book or expert, it's not your Heart's Question. The question may still be important to research, or it may just satisfy curiosity, but it's not one you could "live" or manifest in every moment of your life, with every step inlife, or in the labyrinth. I think of these kinds of questions, which can be answered with "definitely," 'maybe,' or "it depends," as questions to ask the "Magic 8 Ball®," a toy by Mattel®. They include queries such as, "Will I be a good mother?"; "Will I be able to handle the pain?"; and "How can I avoid a cesarean?" Magic 8 Ball® questions not only leave you open to someone else's answering for you "not" doing what you really want to do. However, when you walk and breathe your Heart's Question, you are living the answer right now, with every breath, with every step. (See "Finding Your Question" in *Birthing From Within*, pages 2-3.)

Make the labyrinth a path of inquiry.

Contemplate your Heart's question as you walk.

Enrich Your Prenatal Appointments
with Labyrinth Meditations

W<small>E DON'T HAVE MANY "RITUALS" DURING THE CHILDBEARING YEAR.</small> Prenatal appointments may be the closest thing we have as a modern ritual of preparation. As such, make prenatal care more personal by taking a little time before or after your appointments to practice labyrinth meditations.

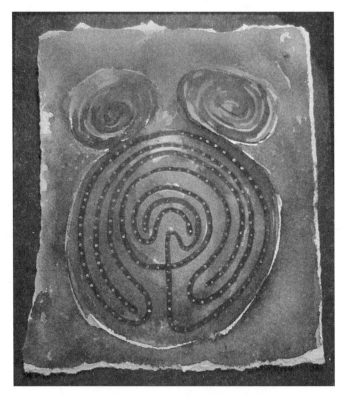

Labyrinth Art by Jessica Deltac

Solution-Focused Decision Making in the Labyrinth

Follow in the footsteps of the wise women of Cornwall who used their slate labyrinths as a tool for answering questions and making decisions. The labyrinth shifts brain waves from beta (linear thinking) to alpha and theta. Thus, using a labyrinth, you may find a new way of seeing a "problem," or discover a creative solution to a problem.

Try this: Before "entering" the labyrinth, sit quietly while pinpointing the problem. Spend a few minutes reviewing all the solutions you've thought of to this point; allow your mind to review and even argue all the pros and cons for each solution. Don't be rational or try to make a decision, just let your mind re-examine the problem. You may do this alone in your mind or in your journal or while sitting with someone who is a good listener, someone who can sit *quietly* with you as a witness to your process while you trace your labyrinth. Refrain from engaging in a lively discussion or "sharing" of problems.

If you are confiding in someone who is a good listener and you have two labyrinths, try this: Both of you set an intention to be receptive to discovering a new solution, while simultaneously tracing your labyrinths. Trace your labyrinths seven times to drop into the "alpha state." You do not have to be in sync with one another or begin and finish at exactly the same time.

What's next? After considering the problem and solutions from different perspectives "do the next best thing."

Make Your Own Power-Animal Labyrinth

ALTHOUGH WE DON'T KNOW IF OR HOW THE NAZCA PEOPLE used labyrinths for childbirth preparation, it has been speculated that the ancestors walked the totemic animal labyrinths to embody the attributes, power, and energies of the animal. Is there an animal you associate with easy birthing or good mothering? Learn about its attributes, how it gives birth, and mothers its young. Consider making an animal labyrinth (of paper or clay), and, while slowly finger tracing the paths or "mirror" lines seven times slowly, imagine embodying the animal's power and mothering instincts during labor and as a mother.

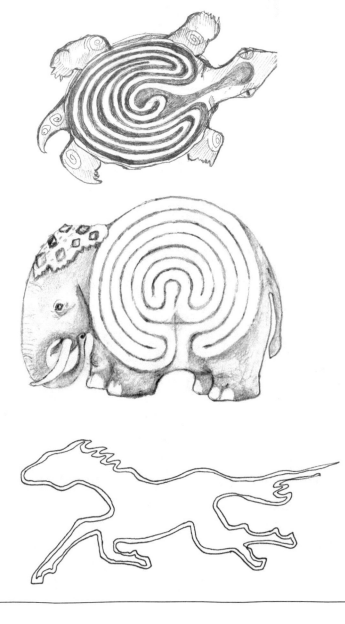

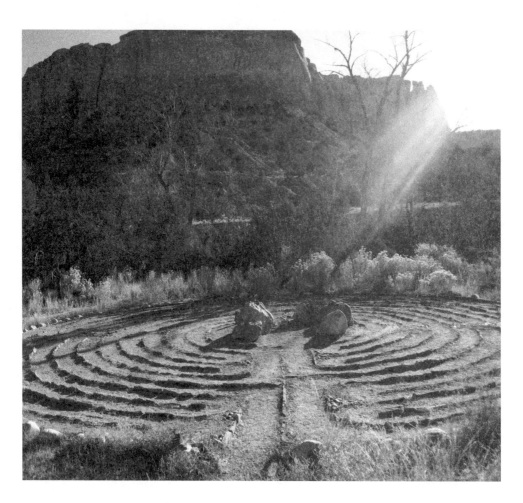

YOUR FIRST STEP INTO THE LABYRINTH IS AN INWARD ONE.

Walking Meditation in a Labyrinth

A LONG TIME AGO, WALKING A LABYRINTH might have been "equivalent to the rite of walking around a temple (*pradnakshina*), or [walking up] the progressive elevation, terrace by terrace, up to the 'pure lands' at the highest level of the temple or pyramid."[5]

Medieval pilgrims walked 364 feet in the Chartres Cathedral labyrinth, built in 1200 A.D. The root word of labyrinth is *labyr*, which means "to turn," and in the Chartres labyrinth, there are 34 turns in the 11-circuit labyrinth. This labyrinth was constructed from 272 stones which, Helen Curry observes, is about the average number of days in human gestation. Perhaps, she speculates, parents used it as an instrument for prenatal meditation, walking it "to achieve good fortune for the child's life, or as a meditation on the process of birth and renewal."[6] Walking a labyrinth enriches ceremonies (e.g., Mother Blessings).

With the renewed interest in labyrinths, you may find a labyrinth in a park or community building near you. You can also draw one with chalk on a driveway, a parking lot or make or buy one painted on canvas. If you have space in your yard, construct a labyrinth with stones, branches, or candles. You can walk it as part of your prenatal meditations and in early labor. Later, you can walk with your baby under the stars—it will soothe you both.

Here are a few ideas to guide your walking meditation:

Walk in silence.
Walk in sync with your breath.

Gaze softly,
downward,
inward

Keep a pace that is natural
and grounding.
Don't watch the clock.

With each step,
recite a prayer
or name for the Creator.

With each breath,
ask your Heart's Question.
Sing a hymn within
so only the Holy can hear it.

FINDING AND KEEPING YOUR PACE

IT DOESN'T MATTER WHETHER YOU WALK QUICKLY OR SLOWLY, but it does matter that you are mindful and regular with your pacing throughout (without being self-conscious or trying to appear a certain way).

Depending on your pace and depth of inhalation, you'll take three, four, or five steps as you inhale and as you fully exhale. You may want to take one step between breathing in and breathing out, and one step between breathing out and breathing in; this takes the meditation even deeper. If you lose count it doesn't matter. Just begin again. Focusing on counting your steps in sync with your breath keeps your mind from thinking. Eventually, you'll become one with the rhythm of breathing and walking, and you'll naturally stop counting, and enter into silence—bliss— peace. If your thinking-mind takes over again, simply begin synchronizing breath with the counting of your steps until you return to a quiet mind.

Slow Walking: One way to slow down the mind (brain waves) and to move into your heart and intuition, is to move slowly and deliberately. This approach to slow walking requires small steps. You will not be taking ordinary, full steps; this interrupts the mind from wanting to "get somewhere." You will be taking half-steps; when you set your heel down, it will align with the arch of the foot that is on the ground. As you breathe in, raise your foot *slightly* off the ground and move it forward a half-step; it should lightly brush the earth as you move it forward. As you exhale slowly, touch your heel to the ground, then roll the sole of your foot on the ground as you shift your weight to that leg. Notice the slight pause in movement between breathing in and out; falling into this space is falling into Love.

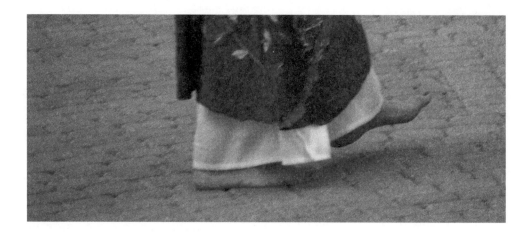

Walking With Your Hero

C HOOSE A PERSON YOU WANT TO EMULATE in your life, in labor, or as a mother.
It could be a relative, friend, teacher, or a hero/heroine you know personally or
have read about. Before entering your labyrinth, contemplate the qualities of this
inspiring person. On the way into the labyrinth, imagine you are walking with and
feeling the desired qualities of your chosen person. As you walk out of the labyrinth,
walk as though you possess and embody the qualities of the person you admire. This
visualization meditation was created by Jean Houston.[7]

Circular Breathing

THIS MEDITATION ORIGINATED IN CHINA FIVE THOUSAND YEARS AGO. In the *I Ching* it is called the micro-cosmic circuit or ovarian breathing. The ancient teaching recognizes that life-giving power, including the power to create another human being, originates in the ovaries and testes. Drawing on this generative power and circulating it throughout the body when exhausted and depleted of energy refreshes the body and restores mental clarity and hope.[8] Detailed Circular Breathing instructions and illustrations are on the following pages.

Circular or Ovarian Breathing is a meditation that can be practiced anywhere you can sit or lie quietly and finger-trace a labyrinth. It is also a walking meditation. You can practice Circular Breathing while walking in your home, yard, store, hospital, or in a labyrinth.

Preparation deepens your walking labyrinth meditation. Before entering the labyrinth, sit quietly and practice Circular Breathing meditation. Without a break in concentration, continue practicing Circular Breathing as you enter and walk the labyrinth.

In labor, Circular Breathing helps calm and focus your mind, especially during distracting moments (such as admission to the hospital). If you feel exhausted, especially toward the end of labor, re-energize your body and mind with Circular Breathing.

Once you and your partner know Circular Breathing, you will not need to be "coached" to practice it in labor. However, when your partner practices Circular Breathing with you, it will deepen your harmonious connection with one another.

Circular Breathing is continuous and rhythmical, once you learn it. When learning the meditation, it helps to break it down into four steps, which are detailed on the next two pages.

Step One:

As you will soon discover for yourself, this works best with a straight spine, so sit up, stand, or walk tall.

In-breath: Imagine, as you breathe in, you are pulling life-giving energy from your ovaries downward and backward along (the inside of) your perineum, and up your spine to the crown of your head (*Figure 1*). It is important to imagine your breath moving upward following the curves *inside* your spine, not outside your body. Attention on upward-moving inhalation is uplifting and refreshing.

At the end of your inhalation, in the brief pause before exhalation begins, focus your attention on the crown of your head or on your forehead between your eyes *(Figure 2)*.

Keep your eyes slightly open, gazing softly downward. Looking up and around distracts you from your inward journey in the labyrinth and in labor. Closing your eyes completely would interfere with walking. Sometimes closing your eyes in meditation allows you to drift into fantasy or sleep. So, a soft, downward gaze helps you "be here now."

Practice this inhalation meditation for a few breaths.

Step Two:

Out-breath: Follow your outward breath, from beginning to end, downward through your body, from the top of your head to the bottom of your belly, just above your pubic bone. Imagine this life-giving breath re-energizing every organ, every tiny cell, in your body. Imagine your next special breath out energizing and illuminating your womb and your baby. Practice this exhalation meditation for a few breaths.

STEP THREE:

Fill and spill the "cup of breath." During this step you will begin to experience the circular pattern of breath: breathing up the inner curves of your spine, breathing down into your body, up and down. Feel the relaxing rhythm of circular breathing for several breaths.

Now, notice the brief pauses between your in-breath and out-breath, and between your out-breath and in-breath. Bringing your attention to this still place between breaths slows down the mind and deepens meditation. Pay attention to this in-between-breaths place for the next few breaths.

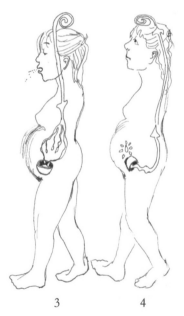

It may help deepen your meditation to add the "cup of breath" imagery. Imagine a little "cup" sitting behind your pubic bone area. As you exhale, instead of letting the breath dissipate, imagine it is pouring into the cup. During the pause between outward and inward breath, imagine the full cup tips backwards and, as you breathe in, you pull the life-giving breath from the cup across your perineum and up your spine *(Figures 3 and 4)*.

STEP FOUR:

Walking in Circular Breath Meditation. Now you are ready to combine circular breathing with walking. Focusing your attention on breath and walking together works like clockwork to deepen your peace of mind.

3   4

As you continue practicing Circular Breathing while walking, you will naturally stop counting and "just breathe and walk" rhythmically. Whenever the mind becomes active or restless, count again for a while.

Dancing Your Prayers in the Labyrinth

*When we fall asleep to the very labyrinth we are constructing, as the making
of our own lives, then we are in deep inertia and will be gobbled up or
frightened to death by the bull-roaring Minotaur that lurks in the heart of the
labyrinth. To dance your dream awake is to grab this bull-man by the horns.*

—www.musicpsyche.org

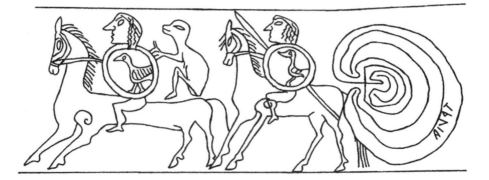

HUNTERS, WARRIORS, AND SHAMANS DANCED their prayers and their stories.
For ancient and modern people, dance is an integral part of renewal and
celebration. It is a profound way to move through and release sorrow and grief.
Prayers and stories are danced in temples and bars, in parades, theaters, festivals,
ceremonies, and in labyrinths.

There is evidence that the ancient labyrinth initially served as a path for ceremonial
line dances. On a pitcher from Tragliatella, Italy (circa 620 BCE), a group of warriors
is shown leaving the labyrinth in a line dance.[9] In the *Iliad*, Homer describes an
image of dancers in the labyrinth inscribed on Achilles' shield: a chain of dancers,

youths, and maidens in alternation, holding onto each others' wrists—"going around with cunning feet exceedingly lightly."[10]

Choreograph your own victory line dance for friends and family that expresses or celebrates your journey through the medical maze of birth or the childbearing year. You may want to do a line dance, because a free-form group dance in the labyrinth may foster self-consciousness and concern about sharing space without bumping into another spinning dancer.

You may prefer to dance your prayers privately in the labyrinth. Wear loose clothing to do your dance. Find music that speaks to you. Be barefoot, if you can. Before entering, begin to move with the music. Lose yourself in the music and in the dance.

Dancing Woman Labyrinth™, designed by Lisa Gidlow Moriarty, tells her story of survival and loss: her and her mother's journeys through cancer.

"The symbolism of the Dancing Woman Labyrinth includes outstretched and uplifted arms that both reach out in a welcoming, supportive embrace and reach up in celebration; wild and flowing hair, suggesting natural freedom as well as the crazy and unexpected ways hair may grow back after chemotherapy; entrances under the arms, reminiscent of a mother's or friend's support and protection; flowing skirt and leaping movement in pure grace and beauty; path center located within a womb or birthing space, a place for transformation, rebirth. The dancing figure rising out of the labyrinth is like a phoenix rising upward or, if the labyrinth is turned downward, a re-birth from the womb-like shape of the labyrinth."[11]

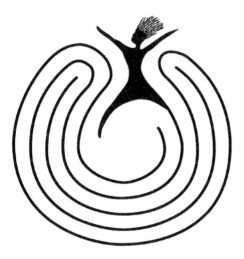

When Lisa's mother became too weak to move from her bed, she said softly, "I just want to dance." Some weeks after her mother died, a young child explained to Lisa that when people die they go up to heaven where they dance with the angels. Since that time Lisa has envisioned her mother doing just that.

"Burning Stick" Ceremony

IN PREPARATION FOR THIS CEREMONY, you will need a wooden craft stick, in which to write your resolution and a fire. You may use a candle set in wide holder, a small campfire or fireplace, or even a special pottery "burning bowl." Your birth or mothering resolution must fit in a small space, so focus on and capture your intention with just a few words or even a single word. This quality, intention, or resolution shouldn't be something that is easy for you to do. Use this personal ceremony to cultivate an action or quality that does not come easy to you, but one that would, by focusing on it, help you mature and prepare for your transition to parenting. Carrying your Word or intention on a stick helps you focus on your intention as you walk through the labyrinth. You may want to walk your labyrinth several times, until you feel you have embodied or absorbed it. Then, upon leaving the labyrinth, drop your stick into a the fire to ceremonially release your desire and prayer to the universe.[12]

This ceremony was developed to celebrate the millennium December 31, 1999, in Macom, Georgia. A group met at noon on New Year's Eve to construct a classic seven-circuit labyrinth from three tons of granite stone. That evening participants (all 350 of them!) wrote their intentions on popsicle sticks and focused on them as they walked the labyrinth illuminated by luminaries, votive candles set in an inch of sand in brown paper lunch bags.

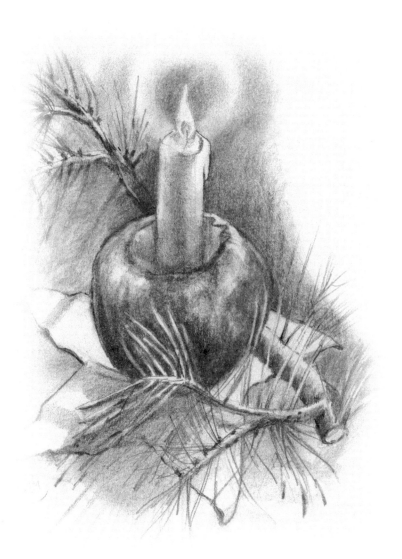

Spiral of Light Ceremony

T HE SPIRAL OF LIGHT IS A WINTER CEREMONY for children in Waldorf schools. First, a spiral path of evergreen boughs is laid down. Gold paper stars are set on the evergreens, one for every child participating in the ceremony. In the center of the spiral, one burning candle lights the room. Music plays while the children are brought into the room, each carrying an unlit white candle set in a red apple. After the children are settled with a story, each child, one at a time, walks through the spiral to the Center.

The children symbolically receive Light by lighting their candle from the lit candle in the center. As the children walk out of the spiral, they find an empty gold star and set their lit candle-apple on it. After all the children have finished, the families sit around the spiral, now sparkling with candlelight and gold stars.

Drawing inspiration from this beautiful ceremony, a glowing labyrinth on a spiral of evergreens or drawn on a sandy beach can become a meditative ceremony for a pregnant woman, a couple, family, a mother blessing or a childbirth class. Variations might include:

- Inviting a grandmother or other elder to hold the lit candle in the center, symbolically passing her Light or Wisdom to the new mother(s);

- Creating a Spiral of Light ceremony to acknowledge the older child/children as siblings. The light and ceremony is for them (not for the baby).

- For a Mother Blessing.

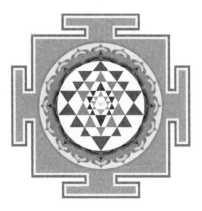

Yantra-Gazing Meditation

T HE SACRED GEOMETRY OF THE YANTRA is designed to help you sustain an idea, intense longing, or deepest question. Yantras are not used to bring about or ensure achievement of a particular desired outcome; rather they focus the mind and remove mental and emotional obstacles.

Hang your yantra (or Laborinth) on the wall or place it on the floor or altar, tilting up the side farthest from you a little so that you can see the whole yantra at once without straining your eyes. To increase your concentration, be still; sit upright, but let your hips sink into your pillow, zafu, or backjack. Soften the muscles around your eyes, gaze softly, and *breathe in* the whole image. Breathe *into it*. Don't stare hard or look at the yantra in such a way that what you are seeing seems to bounce off the surface; try not to blink frequently or close your eyes.

Allow your attention to abide in, flow into, and merge with the yantra or labyrinth. Your attention should not be rigid or forced. Concentrate on the image and allow your attention to flow towards the image, effortlessly; do not think.

Meditate at least 15 to 30 minutes a day. If you practice every day, in 11 days the vibration of the yantra is absorbed into your body-mind.[13]

Yantra-Mantra Practice

The word is a sacred word because it is the symbol of your intention to open
yourself to the mystery of God's presence beyond thought, images, or emotions.
It is chosen not for its content but for the intent. It is merely a pointer that
expresses the direction of your inward movement toward the presence of God.

—Thomas Keating

GAZING UPON A YANTRA IS ONLY PART OF THE MEDITATION. The other part
involves reciting a monosyllabic sound or word called a *mantra*. There are
certain mantras written on a childbirth yantra *(see page 10)*:

While focusing on the yantra, recite a mantra or your own chosen word or
sound on the in-breath and on the out-breath. The vibration of toning the mantra
intensifies the power of yantra meditation.

The word need not necessarily be continuously repeated. Don't activate your
mind by focusing on the meaning of the word. Rather, use the mantra *(see page 10)*
to redirect your mind to Silence, to abiding in the Heart.

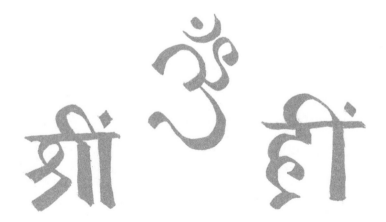

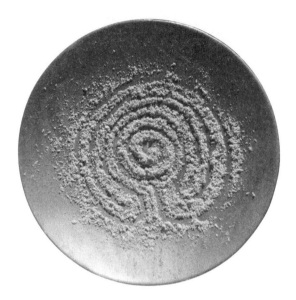

A Labor Ceremony:
Draw and Drink Your Labyrinth in Labor.

Mothers in northwest India have been drawing and drinking saffron labyrinths at the onset of labor for hundreds of years (page xx). You might want to adopt this labyrinth ritual to ensure victory over fear and the unknown in labor, and to symbolically show your baby the way out.

You probably won't be using water from the Ganges (or from any river) and you might not use saffron, but you can make this ritual your own by choosing a powdered food such as (cocoa powder or Emergen-C®) and water, milk, or juice.

Sprinkle the powder in a shallow, flat bowl or pan. Finger-trace a labyrinth in the powder, then cover it with the liquid and mindfully drink your labyrinth as you envision you and your baby finding your way through labor.

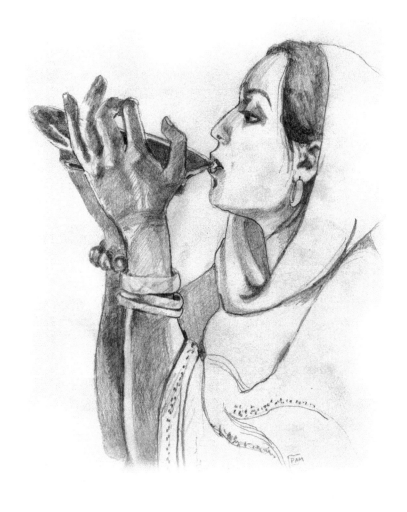

Labyrinths, Death, and Rebirth

THE LABYRINTH IS AN ARCHETYPAL SYMBOL AND A MEDITATION of letting go. It is a symbol of life, death, and rebirth. So, while this book focuses primarily on birth-related meditations and rituals, to be complete, burial labyrinths must also be included.

There are many kinds of death. Death is not limited to the physical body. In a lifetime a human being experiences countless *las meurtes chicatas*, "little deaths;" the deaths of hopes and dreams, beliefs, relationships, careers, and status in the family or society. In the childbearing year, every woman experiences *las meurtes chicatas*. Certainly she will experience the archetypal death of the Maiden in order for the Mother to be "born." The painful death of innocence and trust, a sharp turn in the hero's labyrinth, gives way to lamenting and the birth of a more mature, compassionate, and wise human being.

We are trained by our culture to fear death. Few know how to embrace death as an inevitable and natural part of life, while the majority avoids thinking about it at all. Our culture relies on medical professionals, technology, surgery, and drugs to avoid death at all costs. Still, whether psychic or physical, sometimes death comes during the childbearing year. Babies, mothers, fathers, grandparents, and loved ones may die, even as we prepare to welcome and celebrate a new life.

So much more could be said about stillbirth, newborn death, or the death of a mother during childbirth, and about the grief and healing rituals. In this little book, suggestions for two ceremonies are offered.

LABYRINTHS IN CEMETERIES AND ON TOMBS

In other cultures, in other times, the labyrinth was a part of funeral rites. Often depicted in ancient tombs, the spiral and labyrinth imply "a death and re-entry into the womb of the earth, necessary before the spirit can be reborn into the land of the dead. But death and rebirth also mean the continual transformation and purification of the spirit throughout life."[14]

SPIDER WOMAN'S DRAWING IN THE SAND

When death comes to the stone-age people on Malecula, an island in the South Pacific, the dead person's soul approaches the entrance to the underworld and finds it guarded by Le-Lev-Lev, the Spider Woman. Le-Lev-Lev draws a single unbroken line in the sand, then erases half of it. The dead person's soul has to complete the drawing to be allowed to enter. If she (or he) cannot complete the drawing, she will be eaten by Spider Woman. If the lines are successfully drawn, the dead are allowed to enter the underworld where there is a beautiful lake representing the Water of Life.[15]

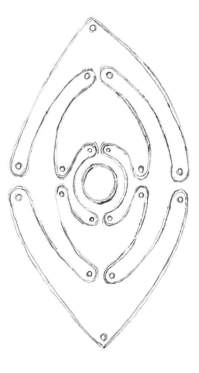

Initiation involves death and rebirth. This initiation myth and ritual points to preparation for death (knowing the pattern before death comes) and initiation into the realm of the dead, whereby only those with certain knowledge are admitted to a future afterlife.

Spider Woman is an archetypal figure found in many cultures. She represents the feminine creative power, weaving a web of thoughts, dreams, and connections within a culture, all from a thread that comes from and returns to her belly.

This pattern does not meet the criteria for a labyrinth. I have included it here because it is related to an initiation myth and because I was drawn to the pattern; I find it soothing to draw and to trace.

To experience this path, trace the line itself. You will see for yourself that, like death, there is no way out. The opening in the center cannot be entered via the path. Perhaps the circle represents the doorway to the underworld or the cave of death, ever open to receive new souls and to allow for exit during rebirth.

A Personal Ceremony: Burying Your Grief in Mother Earth

There is a time for grief, rage, and hopelessness after a loss. And, there is a time for resolution and healing. We know when it is time, but sometimes we hold on to grief because it has become familiar and "alive" for us. Sometimes we are afraid to let go or don't know how. We have been raised to think we can and should handle and transcend our grief alone. When we cannot let go of our grief, rage, blame, shame, powerlessness, or hopelessness, we bury them in our heart and carry their weight around. It is a heavy, tiresome burden.

You can unburden your heart by creating a ceremony to bury the grief for what, or who, has passed on. I learned a healing ritual of letting go from Toltec Master Allan Hardman, and I have adapted it for you.

For this ritual, find a place in nature that you love, and where you will have some privacy.

Look around. Find three little things around the area (a pebble, leaf, shell, or feather, for example). Each object symbolizes pain you wish to release, or whatever or whoever has died (person, career, relationship, or belief). It helps to find a tangible symbol of your loss.

After you find your three symbols, walk around until a specific spot calls to you. Go to that place. Dig a hole in the earth. In your own way, with your own words, prayers, or song, give the symbols of your grief and sorrow to Mother Earth to digest and transform for you. Let your tears fall to the earth. Ask the Mother and your ancestors or spiritual beings for help in letting go. It is an act of humility to ask the Mother to take your grief and pain because it is too great to heal by yourself.

When you are ready, cover the symbolic objects with earth. Walk back to your life with a sense of renewal, with perhaps a lighter step and a more open heart.

In the days that follow, notice small changes in your day-to-day life. This little ceremony won't make you forget your loss, but it may help you integrate it. When grief is healed and transformed, it often becomes the source of wisdom, power, and service to others.

You may have to do this ceremony more than once, letting go in layers as you are ready.

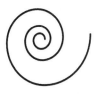

Labyrinth Remembrance Walk

> *A labyrinth marks roads not taken, betrayals and deaths.*
> *On this labyrinth you can mark what should have been mourned in life*
> *but wasn't.*
> —Clarissa Pinkola Estes, *Women Who Run With the Wolves*

If someone, or something, or even a dream in your life has passed on during this year, mindfully make or walk a labyrinth to help you let go. When you come to the exit, as with transitions and endings in life that come before we are ready, turn around, and walk the labyrinth again. Some people walk the labyrinth all night, weeping, letting go, holding on, praying, and letting go a little more.

A mother whose twin daughters were stillborn made many ceremonies for herself on her journey home the first year postpartum. I asked her to describe her labyrinth meditation walk, and she kindly wrote me this moving account:

Sometime around Easter, my mom and I went and walked a labyrinth. It was huge, and probably a Roman-style labyrinth. It took about twenty minutes to walk in, and twenty minutes to walk out.

I remember being calm and peaceful on the way in; I reckoned it to be like a regular mother's journey to give birth. The entrance, the beginning path, was the same that hundreds of other women had traveled during pregnancy and on their way to give birth. I was comforted by that knowledge.

Once I reached the center, everything changed. I was disoriented, sad, and even a little bit happy. The center was where the birth happened, it was where I could be closest to my girls. Reliving the experience of their birth was painful, but it was the last event I had with them.

Eventually I decided to leave the center. Coming out of the labyrinth was one of the hardest things. I just wanted to go back to the center...

After all, it was just a drawing on the floor.

On the way out, I didn't have confidence that I was on the right path, it seemed wrong to me, I thought that I screwed up and needed to retrace my steps. I wasn't lost, I just need strength to keep going. The knowledge that you can't get lost in a labyrinth, and it had to end sometime, kept me going; blindly, I kept on walking.

When I reached the exit threshold, it was unexpected. There was a tight corner, and then bam! All done. I wasn't prepared to leave because I spent so much time worrying about doing it right, when I should have been focusing on myself and what I needed to get through.

I walk to remember you.

The Labyrinth in Your

Body and Mind

Your brain, heart, circulatory system, bowels, and finger prints are labyrinthine. The convoluted tubules in your kidneys are referred to as renal labyrinths. The fluid-filled spiral in your inner ear, illustrated below, is also called a labyrinth.

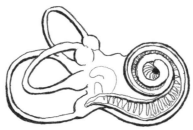

For centuries people have used the labyrinth as a tool for meditation and problem-solving. Many people experience a feeling of calmness and well-being induced by the labyrinth. Midwives and mothers in northwest India rely on the sacred geometry of a yantra to ease pain in childbirth. To fully appreciate why labyrinth meditations work as they do, and to better understand how this is relevant during childbirth, a primer on the brain and brainwave function may be helpful. To understand how the labyrinth manages to have such a universal effect on its users, scientists have studied the brainwaves of people while they traced a labyrinth,[1] with interesting results.

Your brain's left hemisphere is primarily concerned with language, mental tasks, and "getting things done." It is where words are generated and strung together. Think of your vocabulary as a set of tools you use to interact with your environment.[2] The left hemisphere analyzes "parts" and puts them in a logical or linear order; and it is only capable of processing one idea at a time.[3]

The brain's right hemisphere is older than the left. It responds to instinct and emotion and allows you to experience feelings and intuitive insights. Your right brain allows you to see scattered bits of information "all at once," as a whole pattern that makes sense or makes sense in a new way.[4] This hemisphere helps you assimilate the meanings and messages contained in symbols, images, art, music, and metaphor.

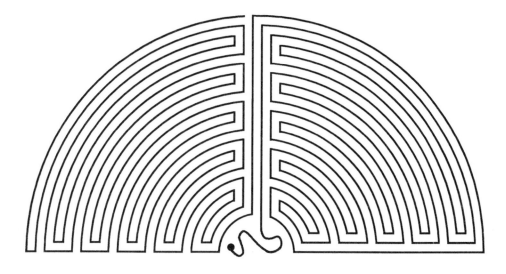

This elaborate mosaic labyrinth (drawn by Jeff Saward, author of *Labyrinths &
Mazes*, and reproduced with permission) adorned the Roman baths in the House
of Theseus in Tunisia. It is large enough to walk. Saward suggests the "thread" at
the entrance might be an allusion to Ariadne's thread.[6] I included it here because to
me it also resembles the brain's two hemispheres and the corpus callosum (the band
consisting of 200 million nerve fibers that connects the two hemispheres).

WHAT ARE BRAINWAVES?

OUR BRAIN IS AN ELECTROCHEMICAL ORGAN. In the same way that a radio sends
signals within a defined frequency, your brain generates tiny electrical pulses
that send various messages through the labyrinth of your mind on four frequencies,
as follows:

Beta brainwaves are produced when you are focused on activities in the "outside"
world during normal waking consciousness; e.g., when you are alert, extroverted,

thinking, planning, or actively engaged in conversation. Beta waves are fast, at 15 to 40 cycles per second. As a society, we favor solving problems by thinking in a linear, rational way, so you could say we're a "beta-oriented" society.

Alpha brainwaves are slower, nine to 14 cycles per second. You produce alpha waves when your attention is focused in meditation, using a labyrinth, creative visualization, or daydreaming, and the waves are stronger when your eyes are closed. Alpha waves create a feeling of well-being and induce calming changes in the mind and body, including lowering the heart rate, blood pressure, and stress hormones.

Theta brainwaves are even slower, between five and eight cycles a second. Your brain produces theta brainwaves when you are drowsy, in a state between being fully awake and falling asleep, or in deep meditation. In theta, you lose attachment to the body, which allows your attention to turn inward; this is helpful in meditation and in labor. Theta brainwaves allow you access to the subconscious and to spontaneously see solutions to problems. For this reason, artists and scientists are often inspired in this state of mind.[7,8]

Gamma brainwaves, typically weak or transient, increase with meditation and intense focus. When gamma brainwaves are produced (25-100 cycles per second) there is increased activity in the left prefrontal cortex, an area of the brain associated with anxiety, fear, and positive emotions.[8] Research has shown that with fast-moving, unusually powerful gamma waves "the movement of the waves through the brain was far better organized and coordinated" in people experienced in meditation versus novice meditators.[9]

Delta brainwaves are produced in deep, dreamless sleep. They are the slowest between 1.5 and four cycles per second. When you can't make a decision and plan to sleep on it, or when you wake up with a solution to a problem or fresh insight, you are counting on delta waves.

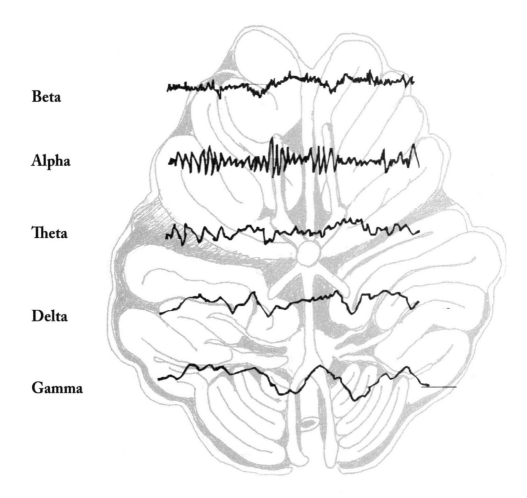

Beta

Alpha

Theta

Delta

Gamma

Labyrinths, Brainwaves, and Birth

Walking or finger-tracing the labyrinth balances the activity between the right and left hemispheres and produces theta brainwaves. When theta brainwaves are produced, left-brain activity drops its guard, which allows the more intuitive, emotional, and creative depths of the right brain to become more influential. Some psychologists believe that when left- and right-brain activities are in balance the conscious and subconscious minds are united. This would explain why tracing the labyrinth (or meditating or gazing into a fire) helps us to suddenly and spontaneously see new solutions to problems.[10]

As a midwife I have often witnessed mothers deep in Laborland (theta brainwaves) identify a problem out of the blue and propose the solution before the birth attendants ever realized there was a problem. This kind of intuitive knowing is not possible for mothers who try to think and plan their way through labor with their left brain and from a limited databank of learned knowledge. For this reason, labyrinth or yantra meditations are invaluable tools throughout the childbearing year and before making important decisions, and especially in labor where they help to override fear and distractions in the modern birth place and create a calm state of mind.

Although I have not found any scientific studies on brainwave changes in labor, I will present my best guess about how and when brainwaves change in labor, based on my experience and observations as a mother and midwife.

Humans naturally begin labor in beta brainwaves. Typically, when labor begins, a mother is alert with excitement and still tuned in to the world "out there." She needs to be in her beta-brain when labor begins because she may need to get home from the market or workplace; if she has other children they need to be collected and settled with caretakers. Finally, she needs to build her "nest" at home or get to the hospital to settle in.

Being alert, conversant, and rational, answering "twenty questions" on admission to the hospital, playing host to visitors, and making decisions—all produce beta brainwaves. Until she is settled in her "birth nest" and turns her attention inward, the outside world continues to engage her thinking-planning-talking-and-pleasing others beta-brain. If this continues too long, it may become a problem for her because women don't naturally labor in their beta-brains. Unfortunately, most mothers and birth attendants don't appreciate how important that is because current childbirth preparation prepares pregnant couples to remain almost exclusively in their beta-brains and to give birth in their beta-brains!

In a well-intentioned, but decidedly misguided effort to help women make informed decisions, modern birth preparation has become lopsidedly intellectual. Beta-brain birth preparation, where the mother must try to think and plan her way through birth, is *contra naturam*, Latin for "going against nature," or "against the natural order of things." Ideally, on the other hand, when we go with nature, here's what happens next:

During mid- to late-labor, providing the labor environment is quiet and conducive and the mother is allowed to labor, she will gradually and naturally turn her attention inward, become less verbal, less social, and more intuitive. The intense concentration required for coping with the increased frequency and intensity of uterine contractions (regardless of method or approach) draws a mother's attention inward; this process produces alpha or theta waves.

Many mothers find that labor is hard work and exhausting. As labor progresses, mothers often feel drowsy or even dose between contractions, helping them produce theta brainwaves. Research shows that when theta brainwaves are present, we identify less with the body. This is exactly what happens in late labor, when mothers become less concerned with modesty, looking good, and even with comfort, as their determination to move through labor and birth their child becomes paramount.

As the shift from being in the world to being in labor deepens, a mother may experience a wordless, mindless, egoless immersion into the activity of labor, a seamless immersion so complete that there is no "I." Rather than thinking "I am in labor," or "I am in transition," she becomes the activity of labor. She may later refer to this as the feeling of surrender; but this kind of surrender is a gift, not something she herself did with her mind. At this point the body truly takes over and the thinking mind recedes into the background. This may be how women, historically and presently, are able to labor without mental suffering and without pain medication.

Is it possible that birth preparation which excessively or exclusively involves reading, research, thinking, and planning—all stimulants of beta brainwaves—could somehow interfere with the natural shift during labor to alpha or theta brainwaves? Just in case, consider taking up balanced prenatal preparation, one that includes both a modicum of research-based information *and* multi-sensory practices such as meditation, movement, and art.

Medical Maps *of Labor*

Medical "Maps" of Labor

EVERY CULTURE USES ITS OWN SYMBOLS and signs to communicate with and direct its members. The Western medical "culture" doesn't use the timeless labyrinth symbol to describe our subjective, *inner* journey during the childbearing year or a health crisis. However, it does have its own symbols, signs, and "maps" to communicate what it feels is important: cervical dilation and time. These signs and symbols have trained all of us, parents and professionals, to focus our attention on—and to fear our failure to meet—timely cervical dilation.

Three examples of obstetrical symbols and maps: cervical dilation chart *(Figure 1)*; labor graph, also called Friedman's graph, or partograph *(Figure 2)*; and charts illustrating the stages of labor *(not shown)*.

The labor graph was initially designed as an assessment tool for birth professionals. It was not intended for parents to see or use. Nonetheless, over the past four decades, this graph has shaped the way medical professionals and childbirth teachers *see* labor, which in turn directly influences the way they describe labor to parents.

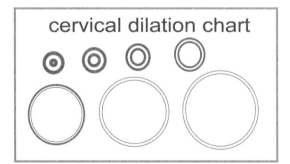

Figure 1

A childbirth teacher might offer an oversimplified, somewhat mechanical and narrow description of labor, e.g,: "Labor is the dilation of the cervix brought about by the contraction of the uterus. The first stage of labor is defined as dilation of the cervix from one to 10 centimeters." As the teacher points to the various charts and graphs, parents learn to objectify labor as merely the dilation of the cervix.

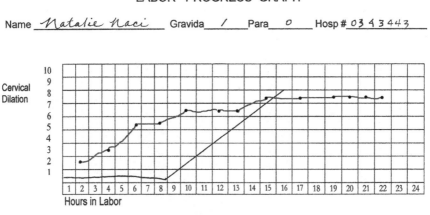

Figure 2

How to read a labor progress graph:

The thin black line shows what an average, normally progressing labor looks like on a labor graph. The dotted line shows a labor that is progressing slower than average; it starts off strong, then slows down, progresses for awhile, then slows down yet again. The graph doesn't determine what interventions, if any, are needed, nor does it predict the outcome of labor. As a visual aid, it alerts birth attendants so that assistance might be given early to put labor back on track and/or to keep the mother and baby healthy.

What Difference Does The Symbolic Medical Map Make?

When viewed as a symbol, the lines on this graph convey the notion that labor, whether long or short, is straightforward. Expectant parents with no personal experience of birth can internalize this symbolic meaning and come to believe or expect that labor progresses predictably or regularly. However, the inner experience of labor is rarely straightforward, and this unmet expectation is one of the reasons mothers may feel lost in labor or lose confidence.

As a symbol, the graph also conveys that the medical model's primary focus is on the birth of the baby, with little value placed on the complex psychological and social *birth of the mother*, or on *her* postpartum Return.

If you are in a foreign place for the first time, you might rely on a map to show important landmarks and turns. If your map only shows you how to get from point A to point B, "the way the crow flies," it will look deceptively simple and straightforward. But if you are not flying, sooner or later you will come to a crossroads, one not shown on the crow's map. Even if you are right where you need to be, you may lose faith and stop. You may even feel betrayed by the map-maker.

If your journey is much more convoluted and taking longer than the map suggests it should, there is risk you will think, "The map must be right—after all, the experts made it—therefore, I must be wrong." So now you can see that it matters a great deal that mothers, as foot travelers, use the right map, and leave the aerial map to those who will be observing the journey at a distance.

Now, it's almost time to make your Laborinth, *your* inner map through labor!

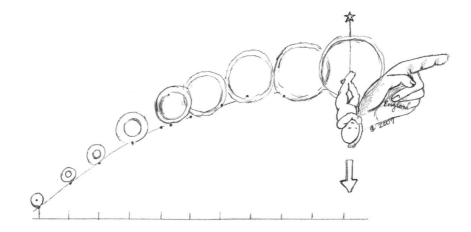

This is the medical map I draw for parents in childbirth classes.

Birth Story

Labyrinth

Birth Story Labyrinth

The soul doesn't evolve or grow, it cycles and twists,
repeats and surprises, echoing ancient themes common to all human beings.
It is always circling home.
—Thomas Moore, *Original Self*

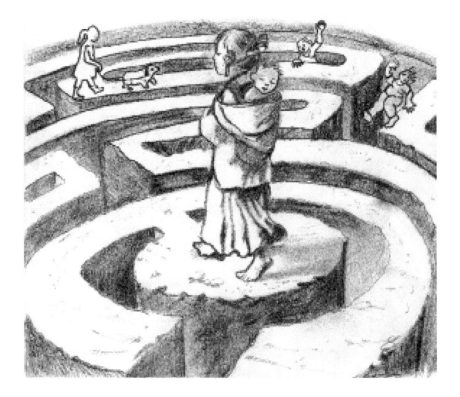

After reaching the center of your laborinth, after giving birth, your journey is not yet over. You cannot stay cocooned in the Center forever, and you cannot cross lines to get out quickly. Just as you were Called to begin your initiation, when it is time, you are Called to return "home" again. And thus begins your passage through the seven Gates of the Return by completing various emotional and social tasks of postpartum.

One of your postpartum tasks is to integrate your experiences during the childbearing year on several levels: physical, emotional, and social. This cannot be hurried. For this reason, most parents say it took about three years to feel they had integrated their birth story and their new role as a parent, and that they were fully "back": body, mind and soul. Day by day, diaper by diaper, step by step, most mothers eventually make it back to the Threshold and step out of their Laborinth.

On paper, exiting a labyrinth is smooth sailing; but living through postpartum rarely is. It is especially difficult for present-day mothers because we don't have many wise elders or rituals to guide us on our way back.

In the first year or so after birth, it can be difficult to know whether a mother is actively integrating her birth story and working through her transition to parenthood, or if she is "stuck." You probably know someone who gave birth five, ten, even thirty years ago or more, and when they talk about childbirth it is clear they are still in trauma. I refer to this condition as being stuck in the Return phase, or "stuck in their postpartum labyrinth."

Mothers often sense they are stuck but they don't always know what to do about it. Telling their story over and over again may not be enough. The Birth Story Labyrinth process is designed to help mothers gain fresh insight which will allow them to move forward, and to accelerate the healing and integration process.

Birth stories are not static; they evolve over time. Right after giving birth, most mothers are ecstatic, relieved, and grateful, and that is the first birth story they tell. It is the only story they can tell at that point. Surprisingly, this is not just true of mothers who birth normally; even mothers whose births were often a harrowing experience tell a glowing first story, one that focuses on what worked or their gratitude.

We hear and read medicalized birth stories in books, classes, on the internet and television. So it's not surprising that most mothers tell their birth story as a fairly detailed, chronological, almost impersonal, account of what happened to them during labor. During the Birth Story Labyrinth process, we break from this somewhat objective, hypnotic story-telling form. Telling your birth story in a new way while tracing your journey through the labyrinth puts what happened in new perspective.

In time, usually a few weeks or months later, mothers often begin having questions about what happened and why. I like to call this "passing through the Gate of Doubt." When contemplating what happened, most women, at least for a period of time, have difficulty accepting or resolving a particular moment during their pregnancy, birth or postpartum. It is often a private moment, a small moment that no one else noticed and that doesn't matter to anybody else but her.

When a mother cannot validate her own experience, she looks to others to validate or acknowledge how powerless, afraid, and overwhelmed she felt. Trying to understand what happened, mothers often tell their birth story to anyone and everyone. By now you know most story-listeners don't really listen to your story because they are too busy listening to their own Story—the one in their own head! So instead of validating your feelings, they commiserate—and tell you their Story. Misery loves company, but it's not necessarily helpful after a certain point: it's just another hook that keeps a lot of women stuck in their Laborinth.

Misguided comments and advice also can become hooks that pierce the storyteller, effectively keeping her in place, in her place, by inducing shame, guilt and judgment. One example is the seemingly universal, shaming, stinging opinion, "What happened to you doesn't matter. What matters is that your baby is healthy and you should be grateful for that." Those words, especially when delivered at an early tender turn in the postpartum labyrinth, are enough to arrest the mother's Return for weeks, months, even years.

Even if no one else has acknowledged that what happened to you was very painful or even wrong, do it for yourself now. The Birth Story Labyrinth process helps you to really listen to your own story, and to acknowledge that that what you lived through was difficult, scary, unjust (or whatever it was for you)—and none of what happened is your "fault." Be still; listen to, and accept, your own compassion.

You can do the Birth Story Labyrinth process alone, with a close friend or a small group (no more than four). Birth Story sessions or groups work best when it's just mothers or just fathers, not couples. Mothers and fathers or partners do not experience the same birth. It is impossible! So, they never tell the same birth story. When couples participate in birth story work, invariably one partner modifies their story to protect the other or to avoid being judged or misunderstood.

I have outlined the steps to follow in your Birth Story Labyrinth. It is actually quite simple, but it requires careful explanation in writing. Take it slowly, step-by-step.

What You Will Need for Your Birth Story Labyrinth:

You will be journaling in the margins of your Birth Story Labyrinth drawing; so, you will need a large piece of paper (18" x 24"), pastels and a pen for journaling. If you are making or using a clay labyrinth, also have on hand paper or a journal, and a pen.

1. Draw a pastel labyrinth, or sculpt one out of clay. If you are drawing the labyrinth, make it medium-sized and leave wide margins all around it for journaling (*see Figure 1*).

2. Draw Footprints about an inch or so away from the mouth of the labyrinth, leaving room to   draw your Threshold marker.

3. Draw a Sun or a Star above your labyrinth. Tether its "ray of light" to you by drawing a connecting line from the Star to your Foot Prints. That line represents the path you've been walking from early childhood—to the moment just before you crossed the Threshold and entered your initiation in the Laborinth. As a symbol, this line or path contains all the stories, assumptions, experiences, and social rules you've heard and lived since you were a child.

4. Journal in the margin to one side of the Footprints your pre-birth fantasy or expectations of what labor and birth would be like, or how you, your partner, and birth attendants would behave, or about meeting your baby.

5. Draw or place a Threshold in front of the mouth of the labyrinth.

6. Journal in the margin to one side of the Threshold about a "threshold moment" that occurs at the beginning of your story, and that inadvertently marked an emotional, spiritual or social transition, or set things in motion. It might be something that happened a day or week before labor; it might the moment you realized you were in labor, the moment your water broke, or your admission to the hospital. It could be a conversation. The importance of

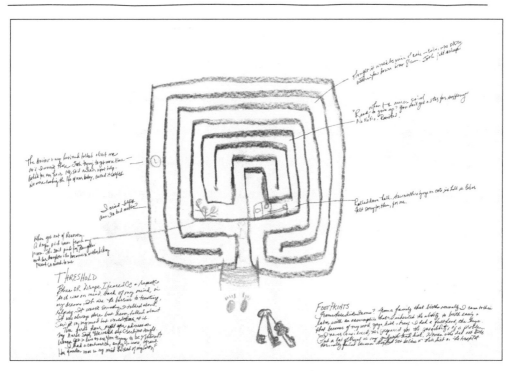

Figure 1: A Birth Story Labyrinth

the "threshold moment" is underestimated. Usually in telling our birth story, we begin after this point, or somewhere in the middle of the crisis. Take a moment to reflect on your "threshold moment." Often, but not always, it provides an important link to what happened later, and how you responded or felt about it.

7. Review your birth story in your mind. It may help to take a moment to close your eyes and watch your internal birth video. Pay close attention to the parts of the Story that stir up emotion, create tension in your body, or where the volume seems louder, or perhaps a part that you want to fast forward over and avoid.

8. Make marks or symbols in the labyrinth's pathways to indicate seven "positive", ambivalent, and "negative" events, conversations or moments, which could include:

> • A particular scene, or a series of events
> • Details about the room, or the time of day
> • A conversation; one you participated in or one you overheard
> • Something you thought, but never said aloud
> • A feeling, either emotional or physical.

9. To help you track your story, extend a line from each marker in the labyrinth out to the margins; jot down a word or phrase to later remind you of the memory for which the marker stands. You know your Story, so you do not need to write details; you do not need to write your whole birth story for this process.

10. Finally, among the seven memories, choose one to work on during the Birth Story Labyrinth session. Lots of things happen during the course of pregnancy, labor, or any life-changing event. All of these moments fit together, and all of them matter to you. Some memories are warm, positive, funny and cherished, while others are disappointing, confusing, even enraging. You can live with the cherished memories, but it's the ones that feel "negative" that you may be motivated to understand in a new way, to find new meaning.

    Using the Birth Story Labyrinth process to bring about a change of heart, you can only focus on one particular moment or event. Which moment? Choose a memory that keeps coming up, that has an emotional charge, or the part of the story that you are trying to forget or minimize, or that feels numb when you think about it. If there is more than one negatively charged memory, choose the one that has emotional pull. Remember, it is often something small and personal; it may not be the most dramatic thing that happened.

11. What are you telling yourself about what happened? What do you believe it

means about you because it happened? It works best if you start the sentence with, "Because [this] happened, I am [fill in the blank with whatever you are telling yourself, e.g., "I am a bad mother," "I am weak," "I am powerless."] In your journal or on a separate piece of paper, jot down this negative belief, statement, or judgment.

We live what we believe. When you tell yourself this negative message, you begin making it true in other parts of your life. How are you living this part of the story, the negative story about you? How is it affecting your relationship with your baby? Or children? Your life-partner? Other women? Your work? Your birth attendant(s) or a subsequent pregnancy or birth plans?

12. Listen to the dialogues in your mind. Most of us are not of "one mind." Our mind is in a constant dialogue—with other parts of the mind, e.g., the Nurturing Parent and the Critical Parent; the Professor and the Drop-out; the Huntress and the Devotee. After a life-threatening or life-changing event, we often engage in a dialogue between the Victim and the Judge.

The Victim tells the story of what happened to her, how others didn't help her or understand her, how it wasn't fair. In a dialogue, the Judge answers the Victim by telling, "shoulding" and blaming her for what happened, for "letting" it happen, for what she did or didn't do to prevent it, for not knowing enough, etc. In response to the Judge's opinions and verdict, the Victim complains more, offers more details and proof to defend herself. . . and round and round they go.

The Judge is the critical voice in your mind that warns and scolds you in an effort to keep you in a safe place, avoiding risks and bad outcomes. The Judge believes if it can blame or scold you, you will learn your lesson or pay a karmic debt, and not let this terrible thing happen again. As Allan Hardman, author of *The Everything Toltec*, says, "The Judge is a Liar. Don't believe a word the Judge says."[1]

When we believe the Judge, we try harder to get it right next time (i.e., the do-over birth plan). Part of us wants to believe that we control our fate and can avoid loss if we just follow the "rules." We want to believe that because the alternative—stuff happens for no reason—makes us feel powerless.

13. Self-love and forgiveness are the keys to healing. At the time this unwished-for event happened, you were utterly immersed in it. You may have been exhausted, afraid, and overwhelmed while having to make decisions. You wanted to do the right thing, the best thing, or perhaps you just wanted to end the intense experience.

Consider this: That on the day you gave birth, at the moment this unwished-for event happened, you did the best you could based on everything you knew at that moment, based on everything life had taught you up to that moment—you did the best you could, and the only thing you could do at the time based on who you were in that moment.

One way to get out of the Laborinth is to cross the proverbial Bridge of Forgiveness. It is time to take the "Good Red Road" from where ever you got stuck in your Laborinth, out…back "home" to your true self. "The Good Red Road" writes Lewis Mehl-Madrona in *Narrative Medicine*, "is the road from wisdom to compassion, the road connecting to all of life from the center of your being, from your heart. It is the road of forgiveness, compassion, and love. It is a road from which we even look our enemies in the eye and shake their hands for making us stronger."[2]

The profound mystery of birth, including how your birth unfolded as it did, can never be completely understood with the mind. Your mind can come up with theories, but it can never fully explain why anything happens.

Cross the Great River—No Blame
—I Ching

14. Close your eyes. Rewind your internal birth video, and as you play it again, notice what has changed about your Story, or the part of the story you worked on today. Notice how you feel differently about it, and what you are beginning to tell yourself about what happened. Imagine your new future with this change of heart: imagine how, when you live from your new belief, your relationship with your child, your partner, family and friends will benefit. Write a new self-belief: a belief that is truer about you, not only in regards to what happened in labor, but everyday. Write your new positive self-belief on your Birth Story Labyrinth, or in a visible place where seeing it will help you to remember it, and to reinforce it during the next few weeks.

15. After completing the Birth Story process, in your day-to-day life, look for small moments, that might otherwise go unnoticed, when your old negative self-belief crumbles a bit more and the new, self-accepting and more truthful mindset expresses and strengthens the Nurturing Mother qualities within you.

How to Make a

Clay Labyrinth

How To Make A Clay Labyrinth

Before beginning, read through the instructions first so you get the whole picture and meet success without undue frustration.

WHAT YOU WILL NEED:

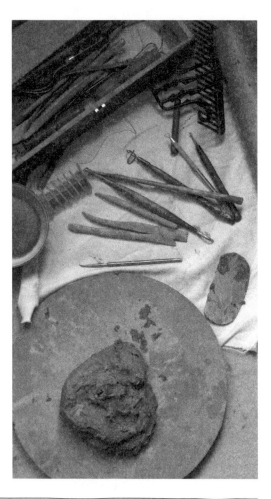

CLAY: You will be handling your labyrinth to finger-trace it during meditation or labor, so you will want to make it more durable by firing it in a kiln. If you want an earthy colored labyrinth, consider using red clay; if you want it in a matte or glossy color, you can glaze (paint) white or gray clay. Another option is to use self-hardening clay. It is more expensive and less durable, but it doesn't require firing.

DRY SURFACE: Roll and carve your labyrinth on a dry, porous surface that the moist clay won't stick to it; e.g., wood or canvas.

ROLLING PIN: If you are making just one labyrinth, use the rolling pin in your kitchen; clay is just earth, it's non-toxic, and it cleans up with water.

CLAY TOOLS: Use the pointed end of a chopstick to draw the seed and lines. Press the wider handle-end of the chopstick into the clay to make even corridors. A variety of inexpensive clay-carving tools—perfect for labyrinth making—can be bought at art, clay or craft stores.

HOW MUCH TIME: You can roll and carve a handheld labyrinth in an hour or two. It takes another week to dry the clay labyrinth thoroughly before firing. If you glaze, you will have to fire your labyrinth a second time, so add another week.

DRY YOUR CLAY LABYRINTH: Before firing, dried clay sculptures are called greenware. Greenware is more fragile than a fired sculpture and will be susceptible to breaking with normal use. Clay must be thoroughly dry before firing. Wet clay and dry clay heat at different temperatures. If the surface of your labyrinth is dry but it is still damp inside, the differences in temperature may break your piece in the kiln. It has to be bone dry throughout before firing. Depending on the firing schedule at the studio, it will take three days to a week to fire your labyrinth. After the firing, your piece has to cool for a day. Finally, if you want to glaze your labyrinth, allow for another few days to a week for the second firing.

KILN: Find a kiln in your community; renting kiln time is inexpensive.

WHAT TO DO:

1. Knead the lump of clay to work out the air bubbles. Air bubbles in clay cause the sculpture to heat unevenly in the kiln and can crack or shatter your piece.

2. Roll out the clay to about a half inch (1.25 cm) thickness. Wait until later to trim ragged or excess edges.

3. Draw the seed lightly on the surface of the clay. At first draw the seed and pathways with a light impression in case you make a mistake and need to smooth the clay out.

Begin by drawing the seed the same way you would on paper. Keep in mind that labyrinths grow upwards. Draw the seed centered and in the lower third of the clay.

4. Draw the seed and pathways carefully. When clay dries, it shrinks, so make the corridors a little wider than the width of your fingertip. The width of the seed and the pathways must be fairly even so that later when you finger-trace your clay labyrinth, your finger will slide through the unicursal pathway easily. If some corridors are skinny, your finger will get stuck or pop out.

5. If you place your clay pancake on a lazy Susan, it makes it very easy to carve the curves as you spin it slowly.

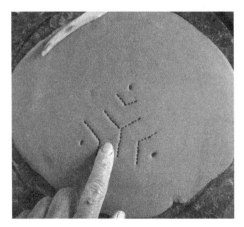
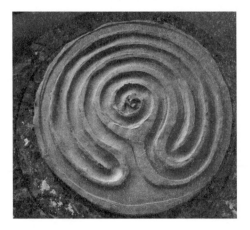

Make a
Sandbox
Labyrinth

Make a Sandbox Labyrinth

W HEN YOU TRACE OR WALK A LABYRINTH THAT YOU CAN SEE, you may be tempted to stay in your left brain: to figure out where you are; to look ahead and make plans; to determine how far you've come and how far you have to go. Your mind does sort of thinking in life, in labyrinth, and in labor—even when it doesn't *need* to, because this is what the analytical human brain is designed to do. For decades, western childbirth classes have misguided mothers by encouraging them to think, plan, and stay rational in labor. Because women are not physiologically designed to engage in intellectual, linear, or verbal activities during labor, this approach to childbirth education has caused countless problems for many women.

Slowly tracing the labyrinth covered in sand, you may immediately feel more alive in your body and senses and drawn into the moment. When you cannot see where you are, or anticipate where you are going next, or assess how close you are to the goal, you are less likely to assess or assume your progress. You stop comparing what is happening to what you thought should or would be happening. When you don't rely on reference points (e.g., preconceptions, plans, someone else's map) you stop thinking you are lost. And at that point you are likely to be more present to the moment.

The mystery of life and birth is a profound invitation to be authentic as you trust and tremble your way through labor's Gates of doubt and fear. It is possible that you will become more intuitive during labor that at any other time. Come alive as you listen and feel deeply with all your senses. Allow your body to guide you in your breathing, in your unique movement, in knowing what to do…even when you don't know what to do.

What you will need to make a Sandbox Labyrinth

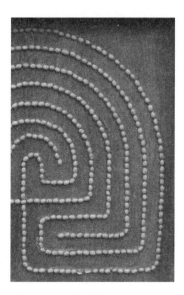

Joanne and Ed Liljeholm gave me this beautiful handcrafted sandbox labyrinth. The pathways are made from carefully placed dry beans.

Time for the project:

- Allow for time to collect materials; an hour to draw and glue the material in place; and several days for the glue to dry before you add the sand.

Gather up:

- A sturdy, shallow box, preferably square, approximately 12 inches by 12 inches (28 cm by 28 cm), or larger. If you plan to travel with it, you will need a fitted cover, like a small pizza box;

- Material to make raised labyrinth walls. Here are a few suggestions: Stones, beans, shells, beads, and thick yarn (so that it is raised enough for your finger to follow under sand), or porous rope or pliable cord (that will readily absorb glue);

- Craft glue;

- A threshold stone, shell, or talisman large enough to visibly mark the opening of the labyrinth when it is concealed under the sand;

- Sand;

- Patience. You cannot rush the making of this labyrinth, just as you cannot rush labor or nursing your baby. Plan to glue a little yarn, then do something else, and come back to it;

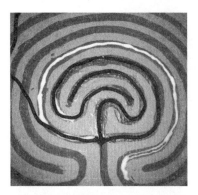

1. Draw a labyrinth on the floor of your box. The pathways should be a little wider than your finger, and evenly spaced all the way through.

2. Trace 4 to 8 inches (10 to 20 cm) of the labyrinth with glue. Press the material (yarn, rope, or beans) into the glue.

3. If you are using yarn or rope, give it time to thoroughly dry in place for a few minutes under a heavy object, like a jar of beans.

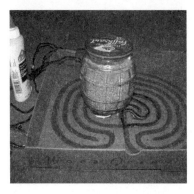

4. Then, taking another length of yarn, repeat this process until you have traced or raised the entire labyrinth with the thick yarn. You will need to cut the yarn at least twice because the pathway is continuous but the wall is not.

5. Glue your Threshold in place.

6. Let the glue dry thoroughly. This may take a few days.

7. Pour sand over the labyrinth completely covering the pathways. Only the Threshold should show through so you know where to enter.

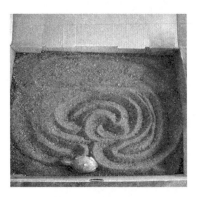

Feel your way through this sandy labyrinth.

Dear Reader,

Like millions of people in the world, I am drawn to the simple, yet powerful symbol of the labyrinth, whose winding paths unwind my mind and reveal endless surprises. I have found the labyrinth metaphor and meditations beneficial in my own life, so it gives me great pleasure to share this ancient and timeless symbol with you.

You have just completed a written tour of labyrinths throughout history, around the world, and within your own body and imagination. As you finish this little book and cross the exit Threshold, you may experience the wonderful irony of knowing you have wound up where you started. I hope you have, and will continue to find the labyrinth metaphor and meditations meaningful in your life.

If you liked this book, please visit www.SevenGatesMedia.com and www.BirthStoryMedicine.com. Subscribe to Temenos, our newsletter and our Birth Story Medicine You Tube channel. To become a Birth Story Listener or Mentor; Enroll in The Birth Story School.

I offer individual appointments in New Mexico, and also long-distance appointments by phone and online. I also lead professional and personal growth workshops for parents and professionals around the world.

Warmly,

Pam England

Appendix

Six Labyrinth Seeds

IT'S EASY TO GROW A WIDE VARIETY OF LABYRINTHS when you have the seeds. On the following pages you will learn how to draw six different labyrinths. The corresponding seed is drawn on the upper left-hand corner or on the left side of the completed labyrinth featured in the frame. By following the basic directions for drawing the classic seven-circuit labyrinth on page 34 of this book, you can draw six variations of labyrinths.

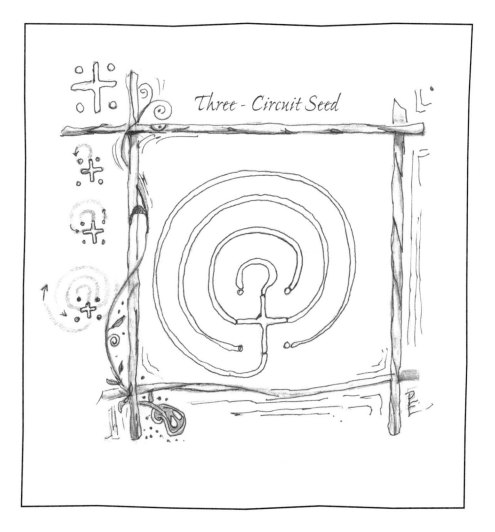

Three - Circuit Seed

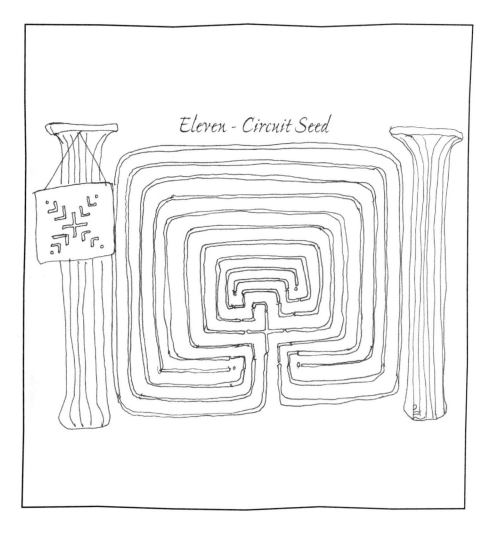

Eleven - Circuit Seed

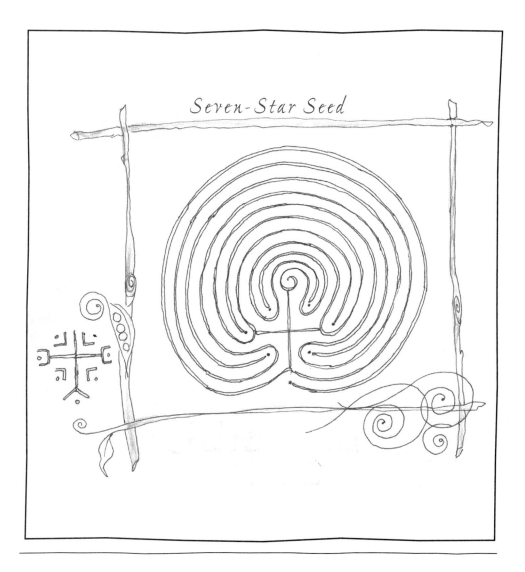

Seven-Star Seed

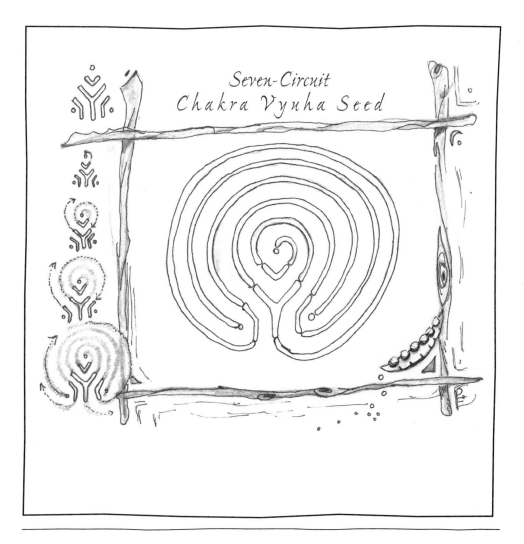

Seven-Circuit
Chakra Vyuha Seed

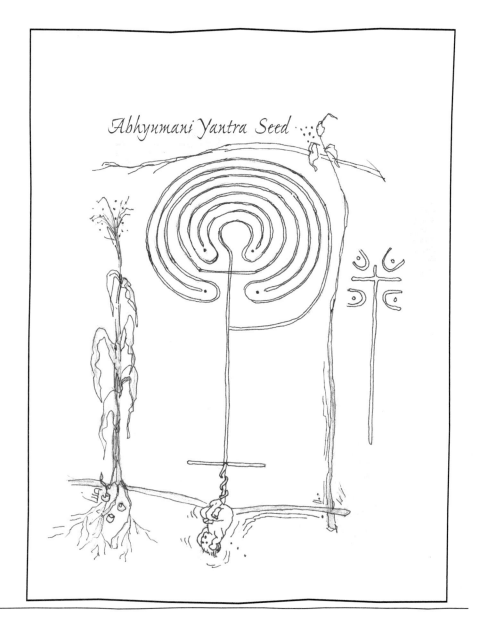

Abhyumani Yantra Seed

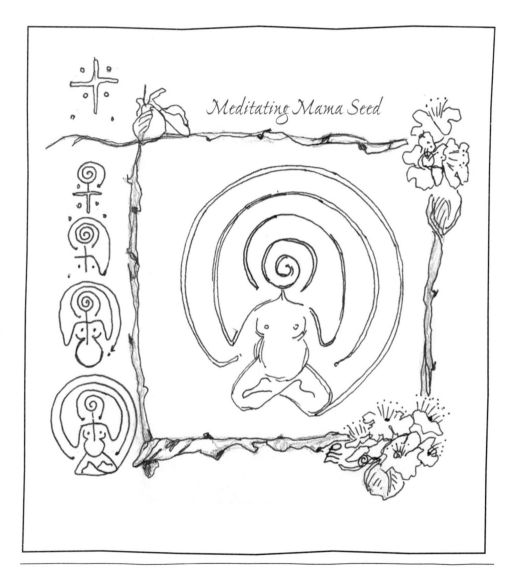

Meditating Mama Seed

Bibliography and References

Special Acknowledgments

I am indebted to Virginia Bobro for her unwavering, generous support of the project over the past year, and for her eagle-eye attention to detail while editing and proof-reading the *Labyrinth of Birth* manuscript and designed pages.

Special thanks to Jeff Saward, foremost expert on labyrinths and author of *Labyrinths and Mazes* (2003), who generously shared his expertise and resources, including giving permission to reprint his drawings of: the half-labyrinth from the House of Theseus in Tunisia (page 87); the yantra (page 76); and the etching on a pitcher from Tragliatella, Italy (page 70).

In gratitude to Mavis Gewant, sacred yantra expert and facilitator, who gave permission to reproduce her drawing of a childbirth yantra (page 15) and offered support of my research and progress.

Soon after learning about labyrinths, Aja Oishi drew several unique rough drafts of labyrinths, including "Meditating Woman" which I fleshed out   nd 133).

After meeting at a workshop, Jessica Deltac from California sent me photos of her birth labyrinth artwork. She has given permission to reproduce the images of the clay sculpture of laboring mother in the labyrinth (page 25) and labyrinth belly (page 58).

Photo and Artwork Credits

All photos and illustrations by the author, unless otherwise indicated; copyright 2010 Pam England.

Page xi "Laborinth: Mother in a Rope Frame," painting by Pam England, copyright 2009.

Page xii Photograph of Pam England, by Sky Tallman, copyright 2010.

Page 2 City of Jericho Labyrinth in the Farhi Bible (1366-1883). The Bible was purchased by the Sasson family at the beginning of the 20th century and is preserved in a vault in Europe.

Page 7 "Family in the Maze," drawing of a basket by Pam England, copyright 2009.

Page 15 "Childbirth Yantra," by Mavis Gewant. Reproduced with permission.

Page 20 "Labyrinth Mama," drawing by Pam England, copyright 2009.

Page 25 "Birthing Woman in a Labyrinth," sculpture by Jessica Deltac, copyright 2009. Reproduced with permission.

Page 28 Re-creation by Pam England of a parents' painting on a rock.

Page 29 Re-creation by Pam England of an original drawing by Marie-Jeanne Girin.

Page 30 Photograph by Virginia Bobro, copyright 2009. Reproduced with permission.

Page 32 "Passing the Seed," drawing by Pam England, copyright 2008.

Page 34 "Step-by-Step: Seven-Circuit Labyrinth," drawing by Virginia Bobro, copyright 2010.

Page 38 "Lion Threshold," drawing by Pam England, copyright 2007.

Page 39 "New Grange Threshold," drawing by Pam England, copyright 2007.

Page 40 "Bear Threshold," drawing by Pam England, copyright 2007.

Page 42 "Meditating Mother Labyrinth," design by Aja Oishi, drawing by Pam England.

Page 45 "Enter Footprints," inspired by the images of the chakra wheel or lotus on the soles of Buddha's feet, painting by Pam England, copyright 2009.

Page 46 "Baby in a Half-Labyrinth," drawing by Pam England, copyright 2009.

Page 51 "No Spiritual Litter," drawing by Pam England, copyright 2009.

Page 54 Photograph by Pam England, copyright 2010.

Page 58 "Labyrinth Belly" painting by Jessica Deltac, copyright 2009. Reproduced with permission.

Page 61 "Animal Labyrinths," drawings by Pam England, copyright 2009.

Page 62 "Labyrinth at Ghost Ranch," photograph by Carly Sullens, copyright 2008. Reproduced with permission.

Page 66 Photograph by Albert Handell, copyright 2010.

Pages 68-69 "Circular Breathing," drawings by Pam England, copyright 2009.

Page 70 Detail of Tragliatella pitcher, drawing by Jeff Saward. Reproduced with permission.

Page 72 "Dancing Woman Labyrinth," designed by Lisa Gidlow Moriarty. Reproduced with permission.

Page 74 "Spiral of Light: Candle in Apple," drawing by Pam England, copyright 2009.

Page 76 Shree Yantra, illustration by Jeff Saward. Reproduced with permission.

Page 78 Photograph by Pam England, copyright 2010.

Page 79 "Drinking Saffron Labyrinth," drawing by Pam England, copyright 2009.

Page 81 "Spider Woman Labyrinth," drawing by Pam England, copied from Hermann Kern's book, Through the Labyrinth.

Page 86 "Labyrinth in the Ear," drawing by Pam England, copyright 2009.

Page 87 "Tunisian Half-Circle Labyrinth," drawing by Jeff Saward. Reproduced with permission.

Page 89 "Brain and Brainwaves," drawing by Pam England, copyright 2009.

Page 96 "Cartoon of Labor Progress Graph," drawing by Pam England, copyright 2005.

Page 100 "Mother Walking Through Her Laborinth," drawing by Pam England, copyright 2006.

Page 105 Re-creation of a mother's Birth Story Labyrinth by Pam England.

Page 112, 114 Photographs by Pam England, copyright 2009.

Page 117 "Sandbox Labyrinth," by Joanne and Ed Liljeholm. Photograph by Pam England.

Page 118 Photographs by Pam England, copyright 2008.

Appendix: All Labyrinth Seeds are drawn by Pam England, copyright 2010.

Bibliography and References

Introduction

1 Saward, Jeff (2003). *Labyrinths and Mazes: A Complete Guide to Magical Paths of the World.* New York: Lark Books, 37.

Anatomy and Glossary

1 Matthews, W. H. (2003). *Mazes and Labyrinths: Their History and Development.* Kessinger Publishing, 32.

2 Gibson, Walter B. (1995). *The Science of Numerology.* Van Nuys, California, Newcastle, 57-61.

Labyrinths From Around the World

1 Kern, Hermann (2000).   *Through the Labyrinth.*

2 Retrieved from www.imelda-almqvist-art.com; and Saward, Jeff, *Labyrinths and Mazes, A Complete Guide to Magical Paths of the World.*   New York: Lark Books, 134.

3 Curry, Helen (2000).   *The Way of the Labyrinth.*   New York: Penguin, 23-24.

4 Retrieved from: www.ashlandweb.com/labyrinth/laby.hist.html

5 Lonegren, Sig (2001).   *Ancient Myths and Modern Uses: Labyrinths.*   New York: Sterling, 33.

6 Retrieved from: www.ashlandweb.com/labyrinth/manmaze.html#anchor710601

7 Madhu Khanna (1979).   *Yantra: The Tantric Symbol of Cosmic Unity.*   London: Thames and Hudson.

8 Kern, Hermann (2000). 294.

9 Ibid, 294.

10 Retrieved from: http://1stholistic.com/Prayer/Hindu/hol_Hindu-mantra-four-goddess-mantra.htm

11 Kern, Hermann (2000). 5.

12 Ibid, 293.

13 Ibid, 293.

14 Ibid, 294.

15 Ibid, 133.

16   Gewant, Mavis, personal correspondence.

17   Reich, Helen. www.labyrinthina.com/mariareiche.htm

18   Lonegren, Sig (2001). *Ancient Myths and Modern Uses: Labyrinths.* 27.

Labor is a Labyrinth

1   Blofield, John (1978). Taoism: The Road to Immortality. Boston: Shambhala, 52.

How to Make Your Laborinth™

1   Gewant, Mavis, personal correspondence.

M editations and Ceremonies

1   Moore, Thomas, retrieved from: www.sthilda.com.

2   Retrieved from article "Labyrinth at St. Hilda's"; www.sthilda.ca/labyrinth.html.

3   Reich, Helen, retrieved from: www.labrinthina.com/mariareche.htm.

4   Eliade, Mircea (1992). "Journey to the Center." Parabola, Summer, 17:2.

5   Kern, Hermann (2000). Through the Labyrinth. 293.

6   Curry, Helen (2000). The Way of the Labyrinth. New York: Penguin.

7   Houston, Jean (1998). Passion for the Possible. New York: Harper Collins.

8   Chia, Mantak (1983). Awaken Healing Energy Through Tao. Aurora Press.

9   Kern, Hermann (2000). 45.

10   Homer. Iliad, (xvii, 590-3).

11   Retrieved from: www.pathsofpeace.com/dancingw.html.

12   Reference to millenium walk from: www.lessons4living.com/millennium.htm.

13   Khanna, Madhu (1979). Yantra: The Tantric Symbol of Cosmic Unity. Thames and Hudson.

14   West, Melissa Gayle (2000). Exploring the Labyrinth. New York: Random House.

15   Kern, Hermann (2000). Through the Labyrinth.

The Labyrinth in Your Body and Mind

1 Barnfeld, Amy. "Brain Waves in Meditation." Retrieved from: www.project-meditation.org/wim/brain_waves_in_meditation.html.

2 Shlain, Leonard (1991). Art and Physics: Parallel Visions in Space, Time, and Light. New York: Harper. 390,198.

3 Ibid.

4 Ibid, 392-401.

5 Ibid, 394.

6 Saward, Jeff (2003). Labyrinths and Mazes: A Complete Guide to Magical Paths of the World. New York: Lark Books, 46.

7 Barnefeld, Amy. "Brain Waves in Meditation." Retrieved from: www.project- meditation.org/wim/brain_waves_in_meditation.html

8 Kaufman, Marc (2005). "Meditation Gives Brain a Charge."Washington Post, A-05.

9 Harris, Neal (2002). "Effective Short-Term Therapy: Utilizing Finger-Labyrinths to Promote Brain Function." Annals of the American Psychotherapy Association. vol 5. Retrieved from www.questia.com.

Birth Story Labyrinth

Hardman, Allan (2007). The Everything Toltec Wisdom Book: A Complete Guide to the Ancient Wisdoms. Adams Media.

Mehl-Madrona, Lewis (2007). Narrative Medicine: The Use of History and Story in the Healing Process. Bear & Company, 46.

READ MORE: REFERENCES

• To learn more about Yantras, read: *Yantra: The Tantric Symbol of Cosmic Unity* by Madhu Khanna (1979), published by Thames and Hudson.

• To read more about Tapu'at: www.ashlandweb.com/labyrinth/laby.hist.html.

• Read the fascinating web page by Maria Reiche, the woman whose destiny and life work helped the Peruvians and the world "see" the Nazca labyrinths: www.labyrinthina.com/mariareiche.htm.

• After this book went into final editing, *National Geographic* produced articles, videos and blogs about the Nazca labyrinths. Here is a good starting place: http://ngm.nationalgeographic.com/2010/03/nasca/hall-text.

• For ideas and instructions for a variety of labyrinth ceremonies, healings, blessings, (e.g., for New Year's Eve, May Day, weddings, and many more holidays and events), read: Helen Curry's, *The Way of the Labyrinth*, Chapter 10.

• Attali, Jacques (1999). *The Labyrinth in Culture and Society.* Berkeley, California: North Atlantic Books.

• London, Eileen & Recio, Belinda (2004). *Sacred Rituals.* Gloucester, Massachusetts: Fair Winds Press. This beautiful book is a personal favorite of mine.

• Artress, Lauren (1995). *Walking a Sacred Path: Rediscovering the Labyrinth.* New York: Riverhead.

• Verlee Williams, Linda (1983). *Teaching for the Two-Sided Mind.* New York: Simon & Schuster. This is an especially useful book for creative teachers.

Great Labyrinth Websites

www.labyrinthos.net (Jeff Saward)

www.relax4life.com/research.htm (Neal Harris)

www.labyrinthsociety.org

www.lessonsforliving.com/poem.htm (labyrinth poem and other good stuff)

www.crystalinks.com/labyrinths.html

Index

The labyrinth and Laborinth™ map and meditations described in this book are more creative tools from Birth Story Medicine®.

Book Trade: Order books from Independent Publishers Group.

Individual orders and bulk discount on orders from parents and birth confrences, go to sevengatesmedia.com or sevengatesmedia@gmail.com

Visit us at www.BirthStoryMedicine.com. Subscribe to Temenos, our newsletter and to our Birth Story Medicine You Tube channel. Bring the Labyrinth of Birth and Birth Story Medicine to your community: become a Birth Story Listener or Mentor; Enroll in The Birth Story School.